X-276
PreK & Up
4 & Up

MW01040386

216 FOLD & SAY™

"WH" QUESTION SCENES

Who? What? Where? When? Why? How?

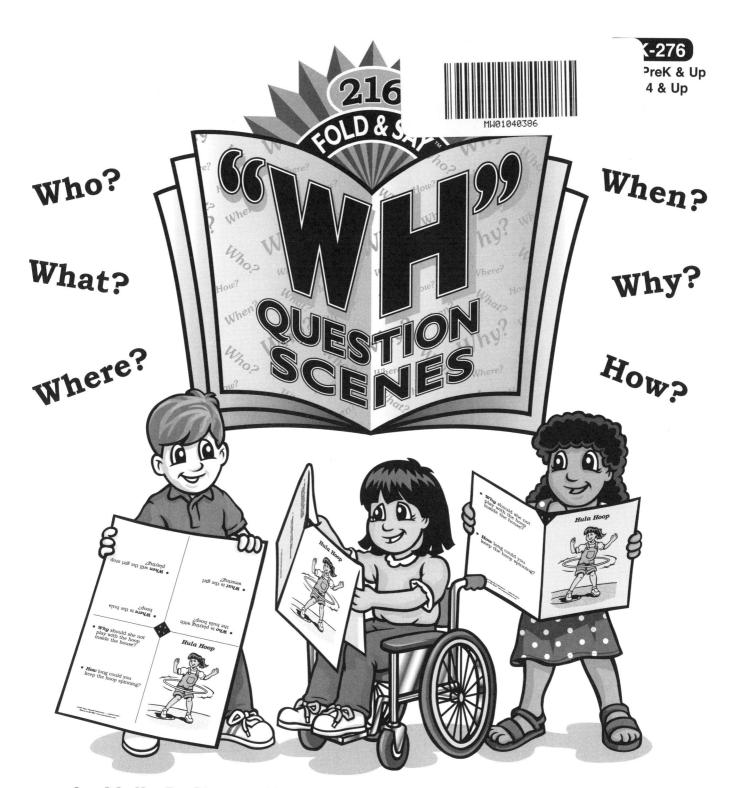

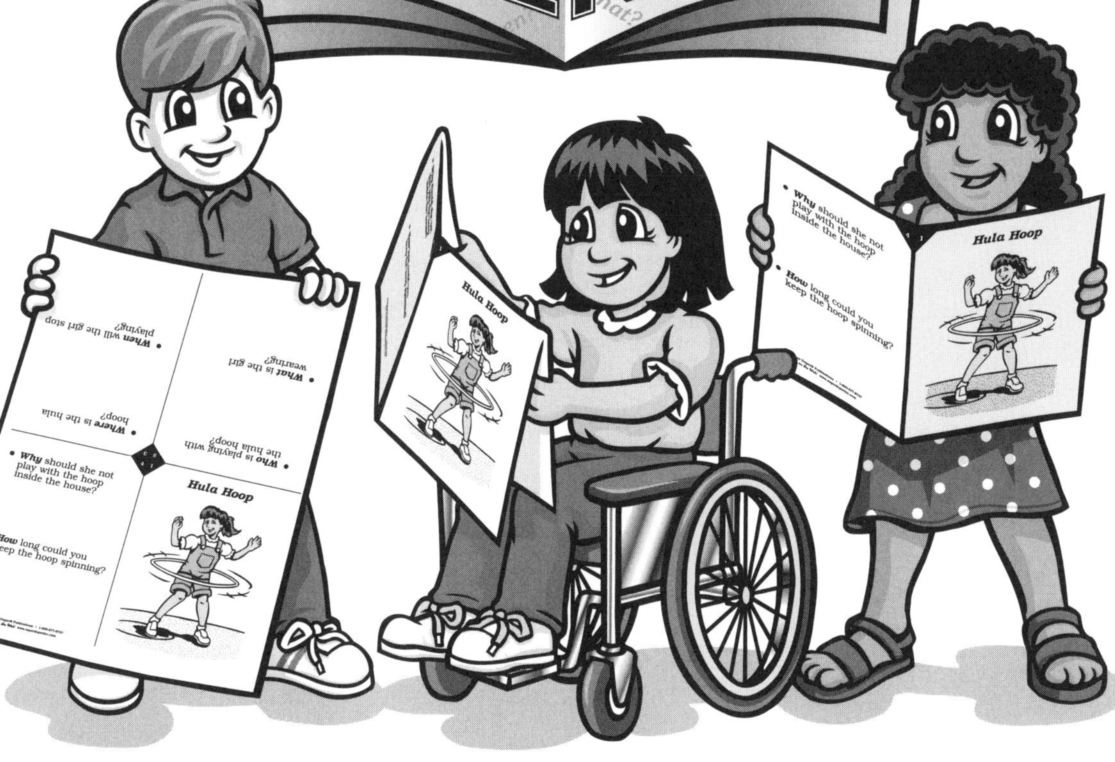

by Molly DeShong, Nancy J. Fulton, and Christina Haislip
Illustrated by Chris Parker, Chris Turner, Chuck Hart & Charlie Denne

www.superduperinc.com
1-800-277-8737

ISBN 978-1-58650-078-8

Dedication

I dedicate this book to my children
Garth and Sadie
for all the times they have asked,
"Why Mommy?"

--- Molly DeShong

This book is dedicated with joy and love to
my parents Mary and Jerome Fulton. Their
wise responses to and
gracious patience with all my "WH" questions
as a child encouraged
a lifetime of learning and growth.

--- Nancy Fulton

To my parents George and Pat Haislip,
I dedicate this book for far too many reasons to
mention.
To the hearing-impaired students
at River's Edge Elementary, thank you
for inspiring me to ask
questions beyond "Who"!

--- Chrissy Haislip

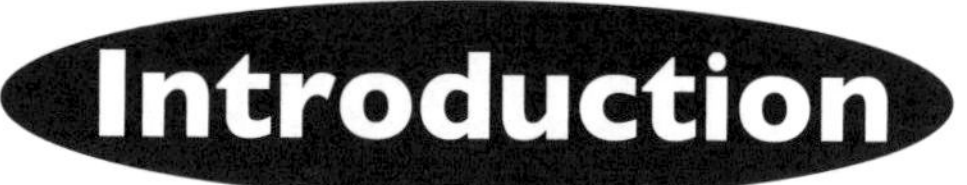

Introduction

How to use this book:

The *216 Fold and Say® "WH" Question Scenes* book is a fun way to reinforce your students' ability to ask and answer WH questions. Each page can be reproduced and folded into a small 4-page booklet. The first page has a picture and the following pages have "WH" questions that will help your students practice their expressive and receptive skills. A bonus "How" question is included on each page for an extra challenge! The book has 216 total picture booklets divided into 12 themes: Bugs, Community, Entertainment, Farm, Holiday/Seasonal/Special Occasions, Home, Occupations, Outdoors, Recreation and Hobbies, School, Space, and Transportation. We have also included a blank *Fold and Say®* booklet in the appendix (page 230) so that you can customize a booklet for your students or have the student create one!

The parent letter (page vi) informs parents of your therapy goals and instructs them how to practice at home. The letter can be signed and returned as the homework sheet so that the student may keep the booklet at home for further practice. There is additional space on the parent letter for you to write in the therapy activities that best suit the student's needs or your own personal teaching style. The following are suggested activities for your therapy sessions:

1. Look at the picture with the student. Read the question aloud emphasizing the question word and have him or her answer it aloud.
2. Have the student write down answers in the space below the question in the booklet. When complete, review the answers with the student.
3. Have the student look at the picture and then answer the questions from memory.
4. Have the students take turns reading one question and having another student answer. Help the students decide whether the answer is appropriate.
5. Ask the child to come up with another "WH" and "How" question for each one.
6. Focus on one "WH" or "How" question and have the student come up with 3 more questions for the picture.
7. Give the student a blank *Fold and Say®* page. Have him or her cut out a picture from a magazine or draw a picture and then write questions. The students can swap booklets and have their classmates answer the questions.
8. Switch roles with the student and pretend he or she is the teacher. The student poses the question to you and you give an answer. To "test" the student, answer some of the questions inappropriately. (For example, if the question is "When do you go to bed?" you might say, "I sleep on a bunk bed.") He or she decides whether your answer is appropriate.

Table of Contents

Outdoors 127-138

Recreation and Hobbies....... 139-192

School.......... 193-212

Space 213-220

Transportation 221-228

Appendix 229-232

Date ____________________

Dear Parent/Helper:

We are working on your child's ability to ask and answer WH questions in speech and language class. You can help with your child's progress by doing these activities at home. The *216 Fold and Say® "WH" Question Scenes* book is a fun way to practice hearing a question and identifying whether the needed answer is a person (i.e. a "Who" question), an object (i.e. a "What" question) or a place (i.e. a "Where" question), etc. Please work on the activities with a ☑ in the box.

- ❑ Look at the picture with your child. Read the question aloud emphasizing the question word and have him or her answer it aloud.
- ❑ Have your child write down answers in the space below the question in the booklet. When complete, review the answers with your child.
- ❑ Have the student look at the picture and then answer the questions from memory.
- ❑ Ask the child to come up with another "WH" and "How" question for each one.
- ❑ Focus on one "WH" or "How" question and have the child come up with 3 more questions for the picture.
- ❑ Use the blank Fold and Say page to encourage your child to write his or her own book by cutting out a picture from a magazine or drawing a picture. Help your child come up with "WH" questions and then talk about appropriate answers.
- ❑ Switch roles with the child and pretend he or she is the teacher. The student poses the question to you and you give an answer. To "test" the student, answer some of the questions inappropriately. (For example, if the question is "When do you go to bed?" you might say, "I sleep on a bunk bed.") He or she decides whether your answer is appropriate.
- ❑ ____
____
____

Please sign and return on ____________________ .

Thank you for your support!

____________________	____________________
Name	**Parent/Helper Signature**
____________________	____________________
Speech - Language Pathologist	**Date**

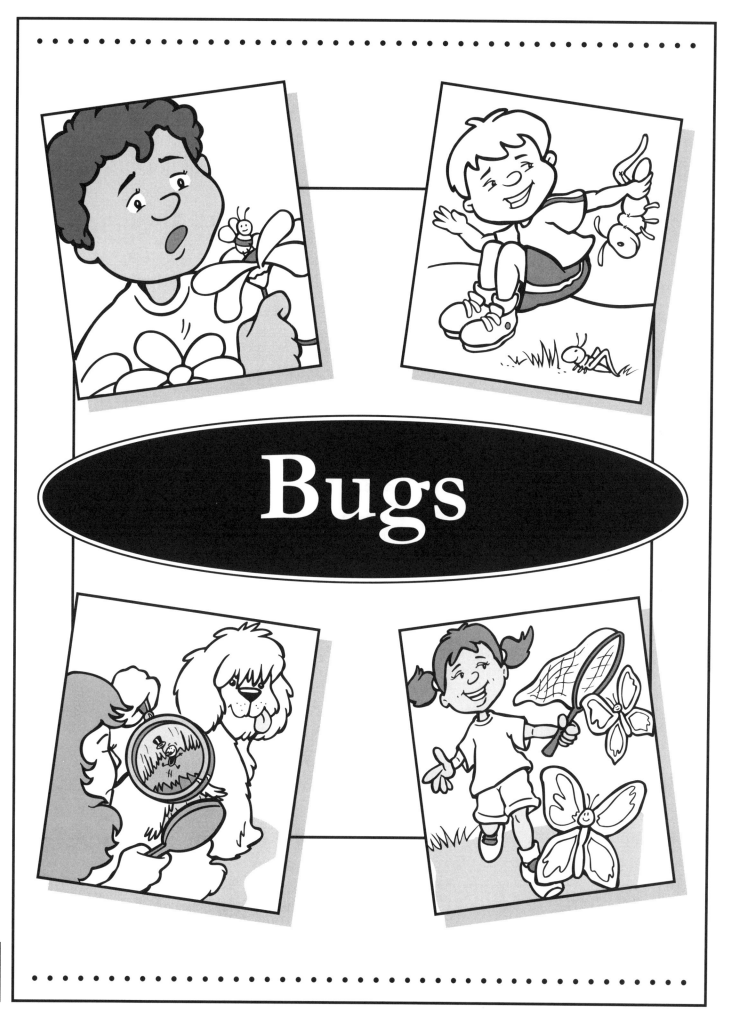
Bugs

Ants

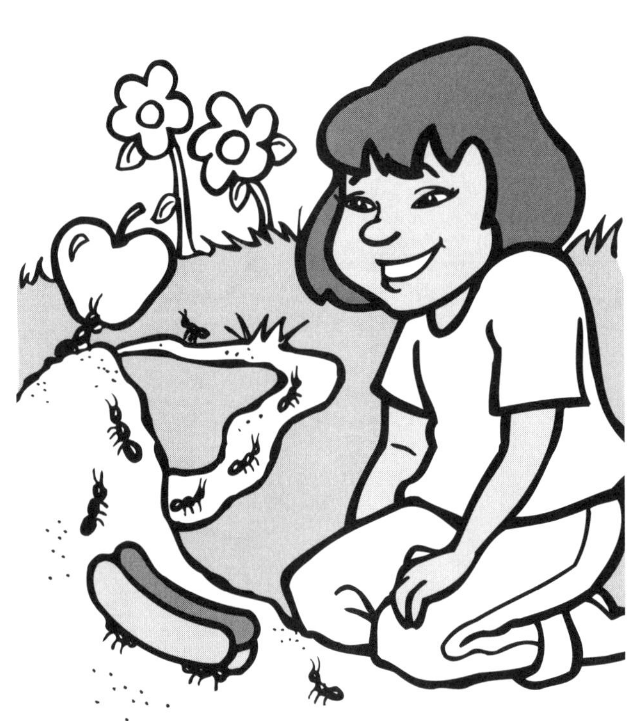

- ***Who*** is watching the ants?
- ***What*** are the ants carrying?
- ***Where*** do ants live?
- ***When*** do ants work?
- ***Why*** do ants carry food home?
- ***How*** do ants work together?

1 2 3 4

Cut on dotted line

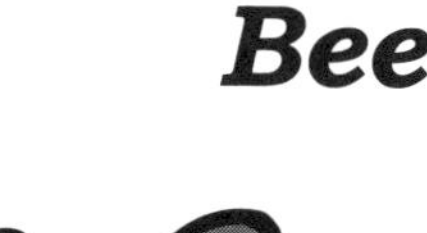

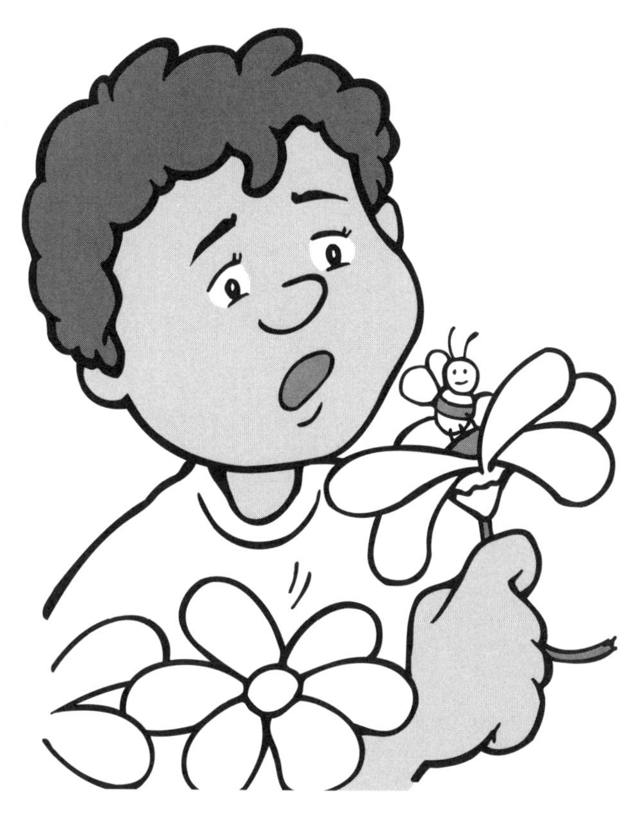

- ***Who*** is looking at the bee?
- ***What*** is the boy saying to the bee?

- ***Where*** is the bee sitting?
- ***When*** do bees buzz?

- ***Why*** do bees like flowers?
- ***How*** do bees fly?

Cut on dotted line

Bugs

Butterflies

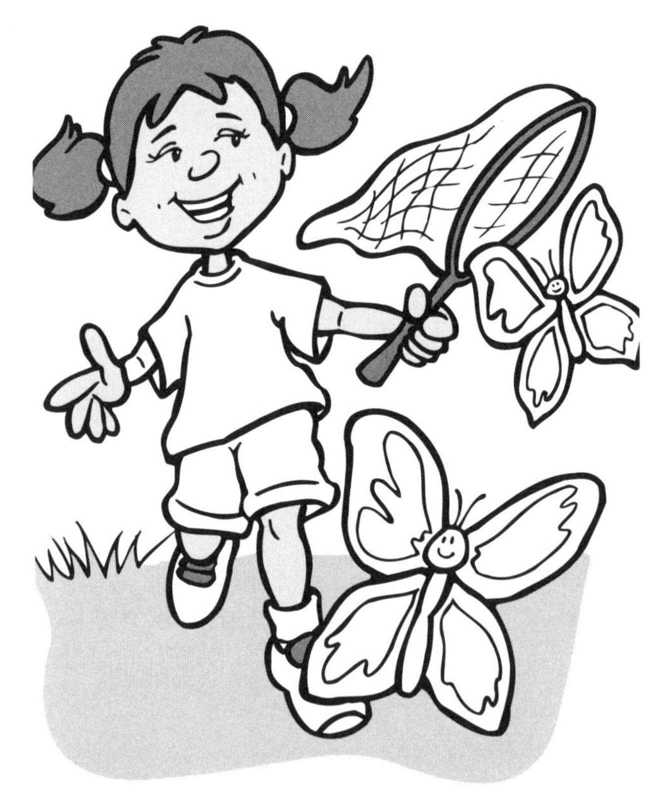

1 2 3 4

- ***Who*** is chasing the butterfly?
- ***What*** is she holding?
- ***Where*** are the butterflies?
- ***When*** do you see butterflies?
- ***Why*** is she chasing the butterflies?
- ***How*** do you catch a butterfly?

Cut on dotted line

Caterpillar

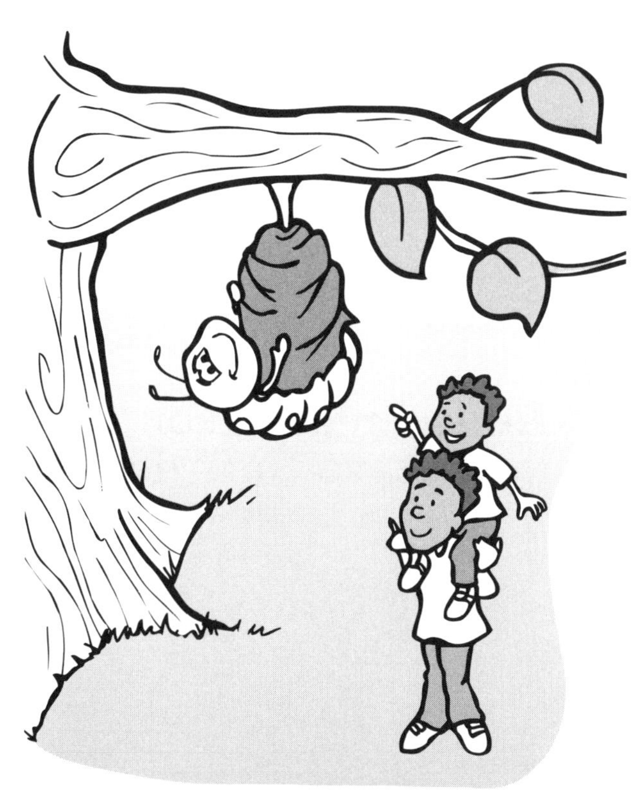

- ***Why*** are caterpillars sometimes found in trees?

- ***How*** did the boy get close to the caterpillar?

- ***Who*** is pointing at the caterpillar?

- ***What*** is above the caterpillar?

- ***Where*** do caterpillars live?

- ***When*** do caterpillars make a cocoon?

1 4 2 3

Bugs

Cut on dotted line

Flea

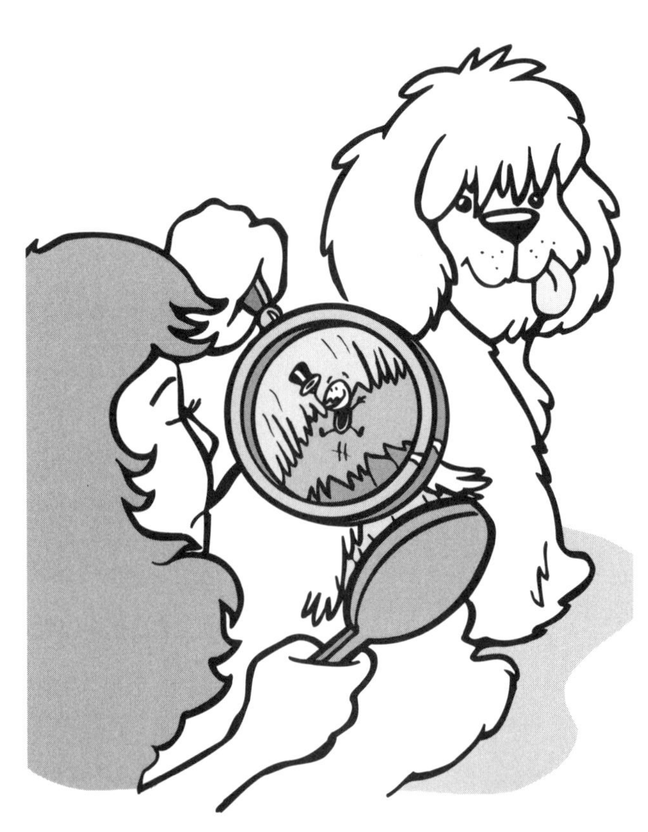

1 2 3 4

- ***Who*** is brushing the dog?
- ***What*** did the lady find on the dog?

- ***Where*** do fleas live?
- ***When*** do people check dogs for fleas?

- ***Why*** do people brush their dogs' hair?
- ***How*** can a person make fleas leave their dogs?

Cut on dotted line

Flies

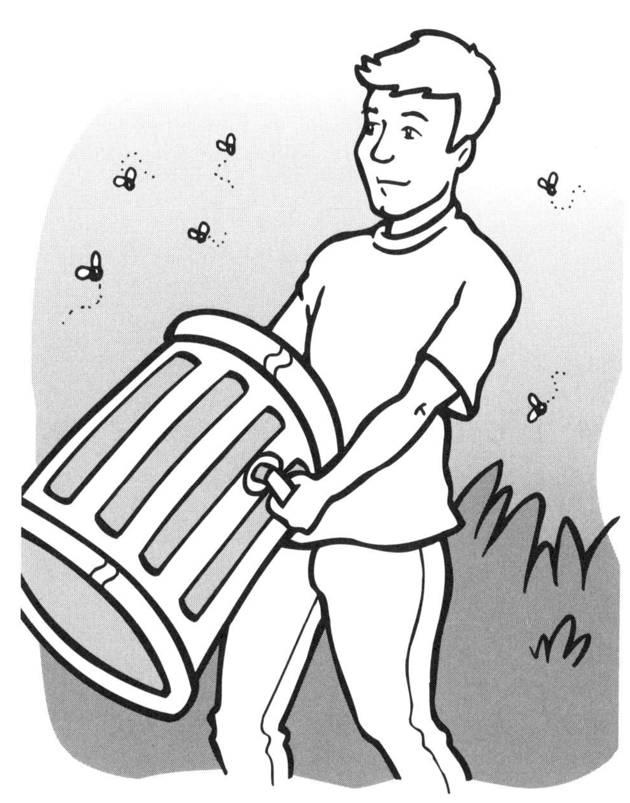

1 2 3 4

- ***Who*** is flying around the man?
- ***What*** do the flies want?

- ***Where*** do flies like to live?
- ***When*** do flies eat?

- ***Why*** do flies like trash?
- ***How*** do flies travel from place to place?

Grasshoppers

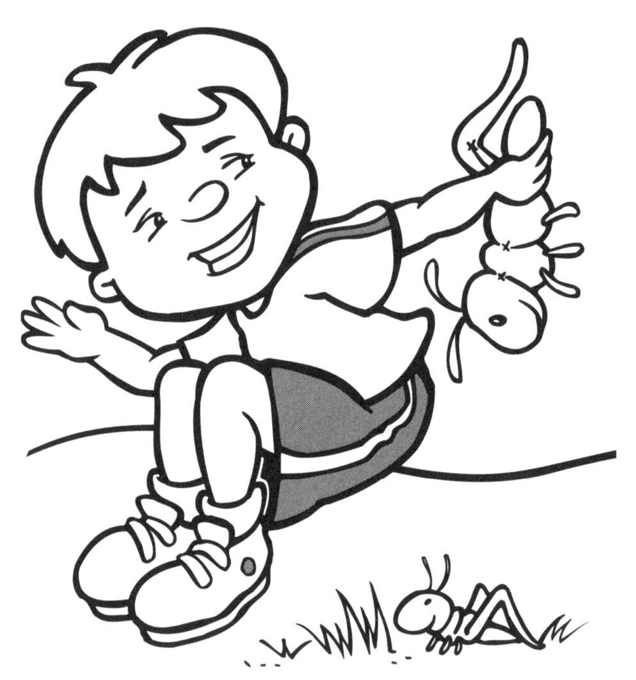

1 2 3 4

- ***Who*** is jumping in the air?
- ***What*** kind of bug is the boy holding?
- ***Where*** can you find a grasshopper?
- ***When*** do grasshoppers jump?
- ***Why*** did the boy jump over the grasshopper?
- ***How*** do grasshoppers find food to eat?

Cut on dotted line

1 2 3 4

Spider

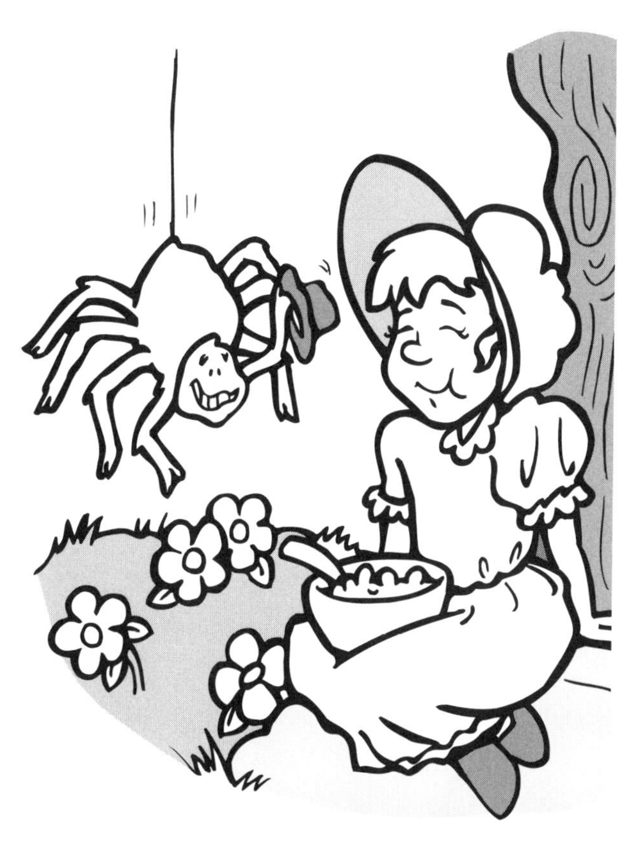

- ***Who*** is sitting near the tree?
- ***What*** is coming down next to the girl?

- ***Where*** is the girl sitting?
- ***When*** do people eat outside?

- ***Why*** is the spider smiling?

- ***How*** did the spider get his hat?

Worm

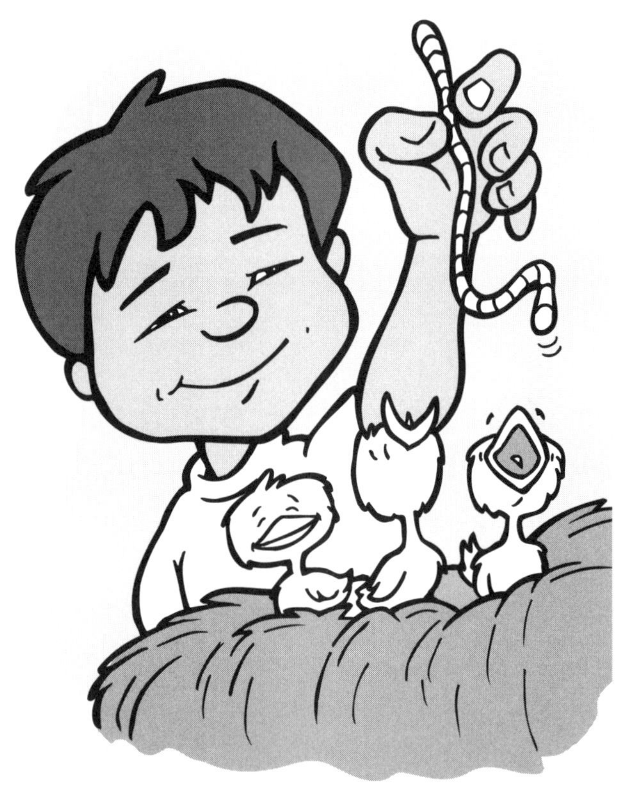

- ***Who*** is feeding the birds?
- ***What*** is the boy feeding the birds?
- ***Where*** are the birds?
- ***When*** do baby birds chirp?
- ***Why*** is the child holding the worm over the birds?
- ***How*** do you know if a baby bird is hungry?

Cut on dotted line

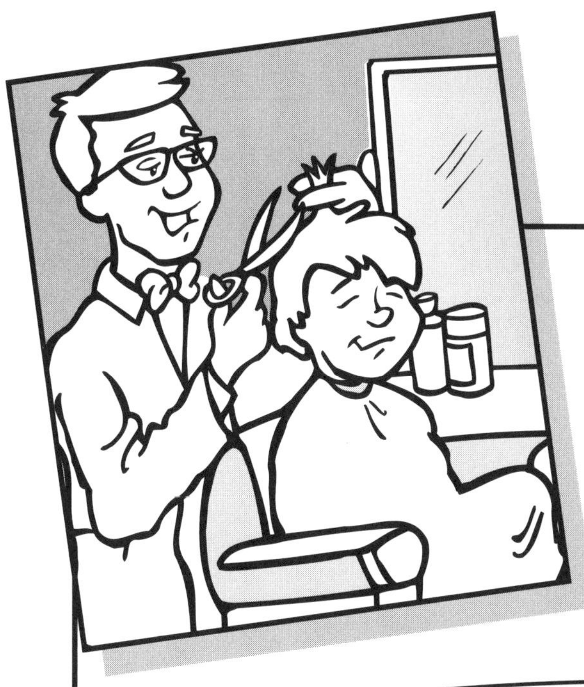

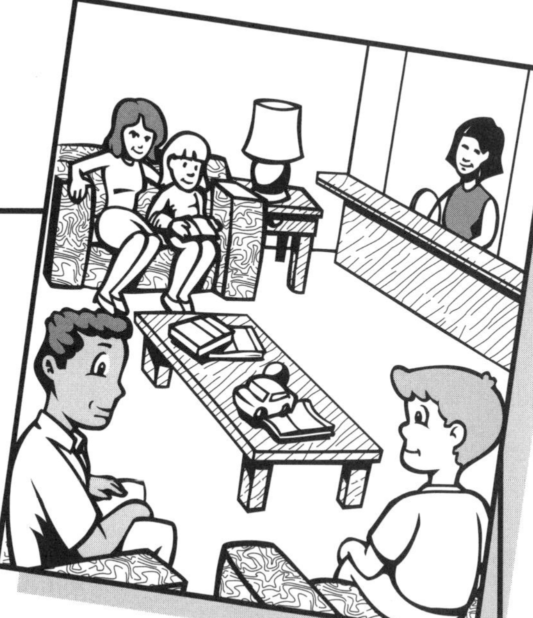

Community

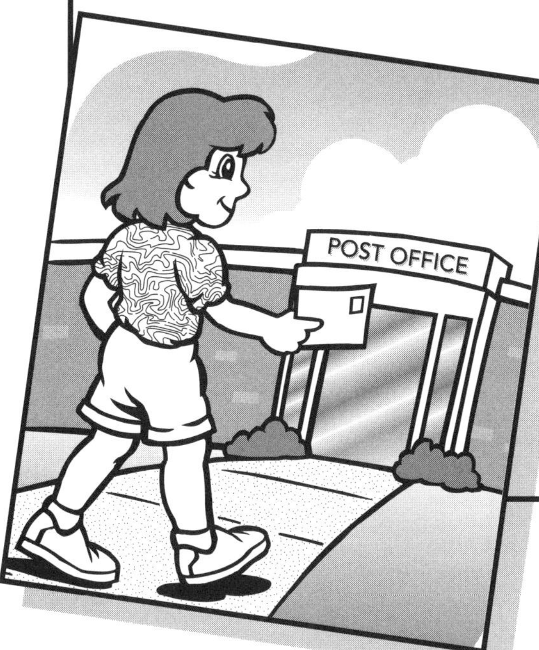

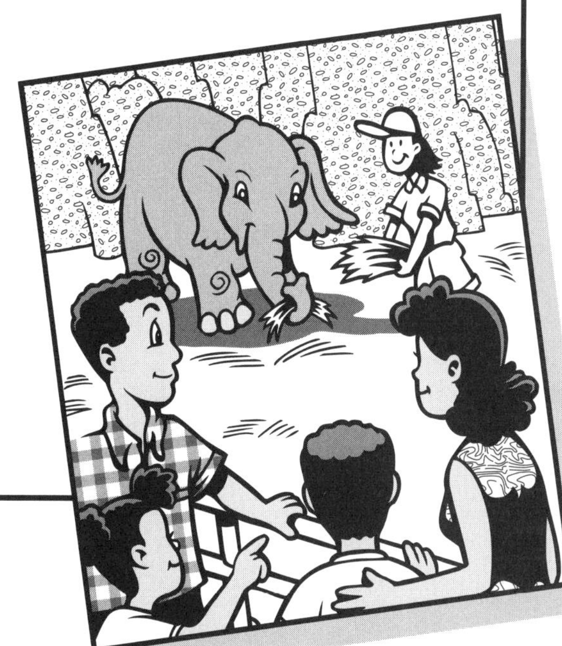

Airplane

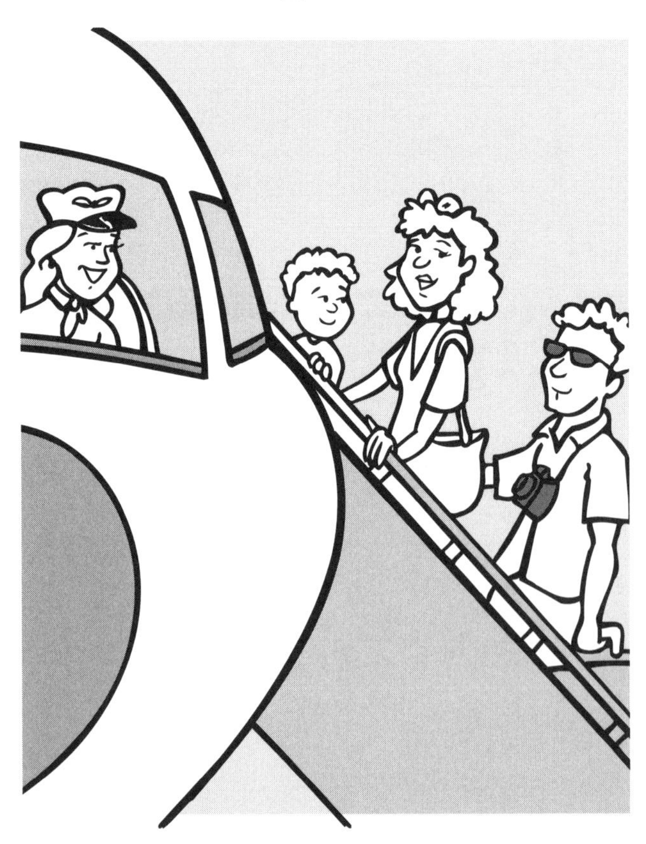

1 2 3 4

- ***Who*** will fly the airplane?
- ***What*** would you bring on an airplane trip?

- ***Where*** does a plane take-off and land?
- ***When*** do people get their luggage?

- ***Why*** do some people drive instead of fly?
- ***How*** high will this airplane fly?

Cut on dotted line

Cut on dotted line

Barber

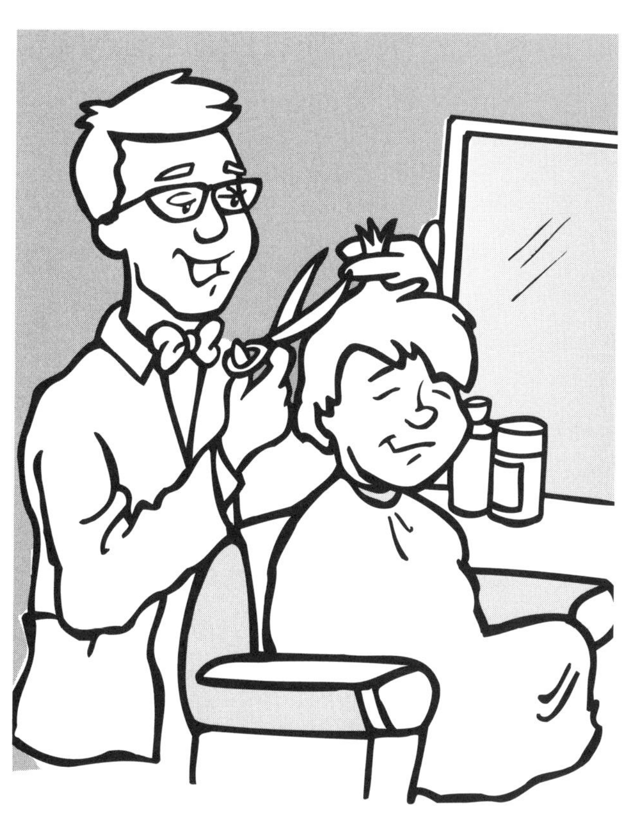

- ***Who*** is cutting the boy's hair?
- ***What*** is the man using to cut the boy's hair?

- ***Where*** is the boy?
- ***When*** does the boy get his hair cut?

- ***Why*** is the boy wearing a cape over his clothes?
- ***How*** will the boy look when he is done?

1 2 3 4

Cut on dotted line

Candy Shop

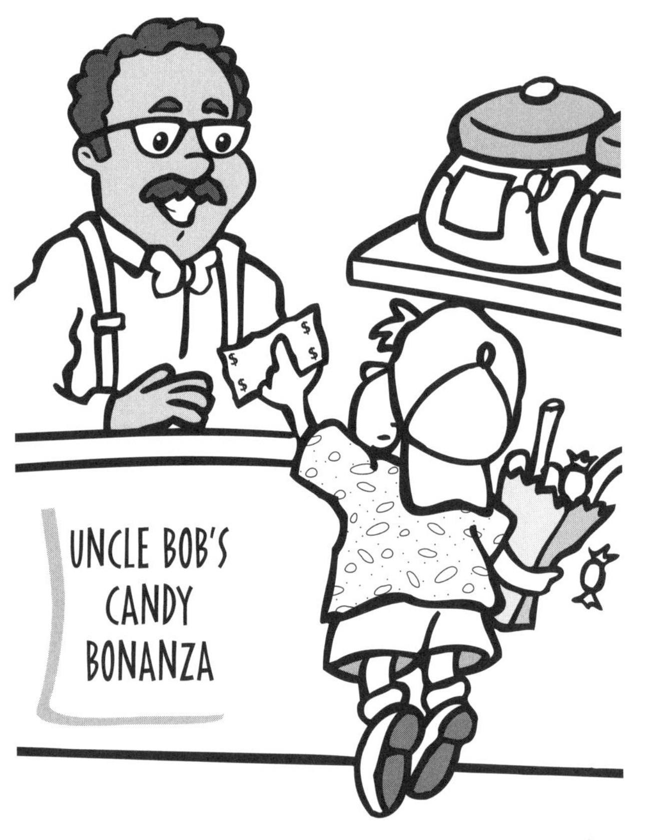

- ***Who*** is buying candy?
- ***What*** is the boy carrying in his hands?
- ***Where*** is the man?
- ***When*** do people pay for their candy?
- ***Why*** is the boy standing on his toes?
- ***How*** long will it take for the boy to finish all of his candy?

Cut on dotted line

Community

Car Garage

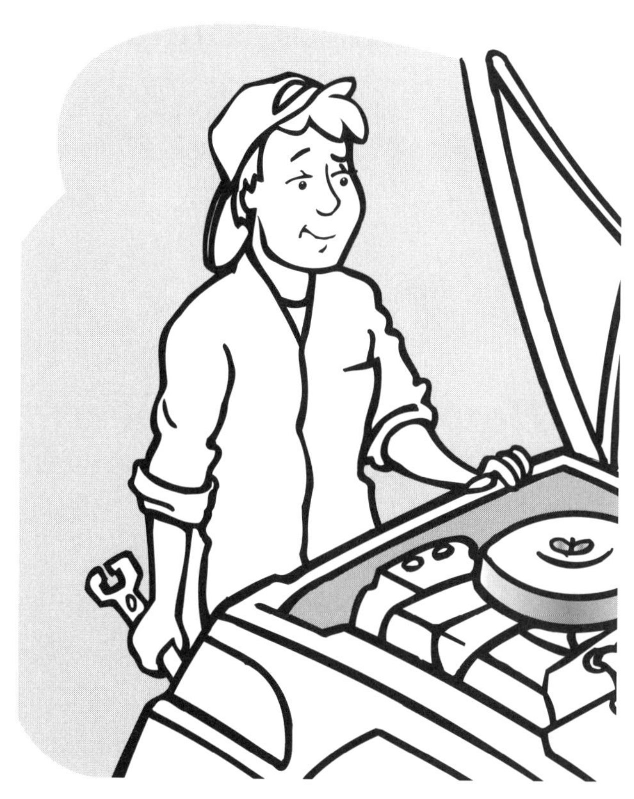

- ***Who*** fixes a car when it is broken?
- ***What*** is wrong with this car?

- ***Where*** do people take cars to be repaired?
- ***When*** did the car break down?

- ***Why*** do people use cars?
- ***How*** can you tell if a car is broken?

Cut on dotted line

Community

Page 16

Car Wash

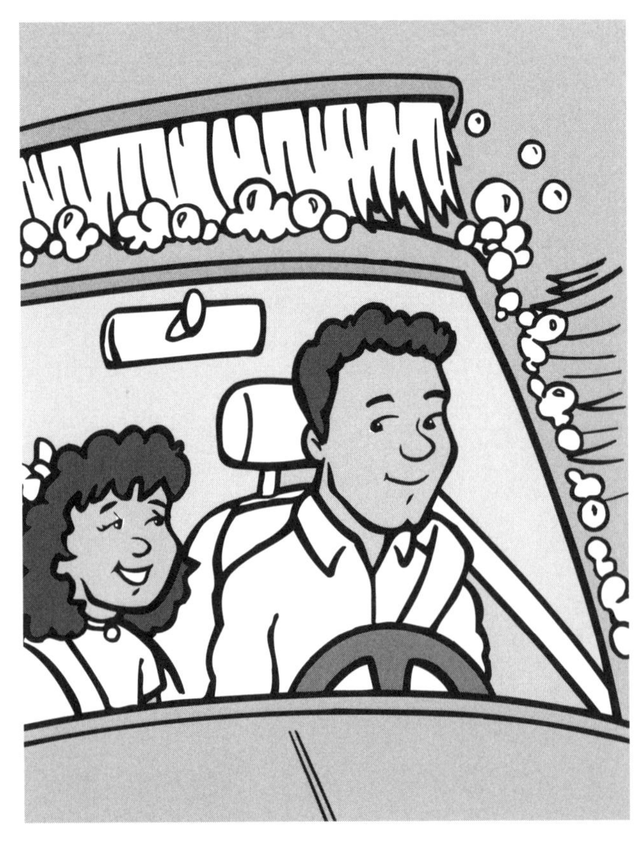

1 2 3 4

- ***Who*** drives the car through the wash?
- ***What*** washes the dirt off the car?

- ***Where*** are the man and the girl?
- ***When*** should a car be washed?

- ***Why*** do some people wash cars by hand?
- ***How*** long will the car wash take?

Cut on dotted line

Community

Dentist's Office

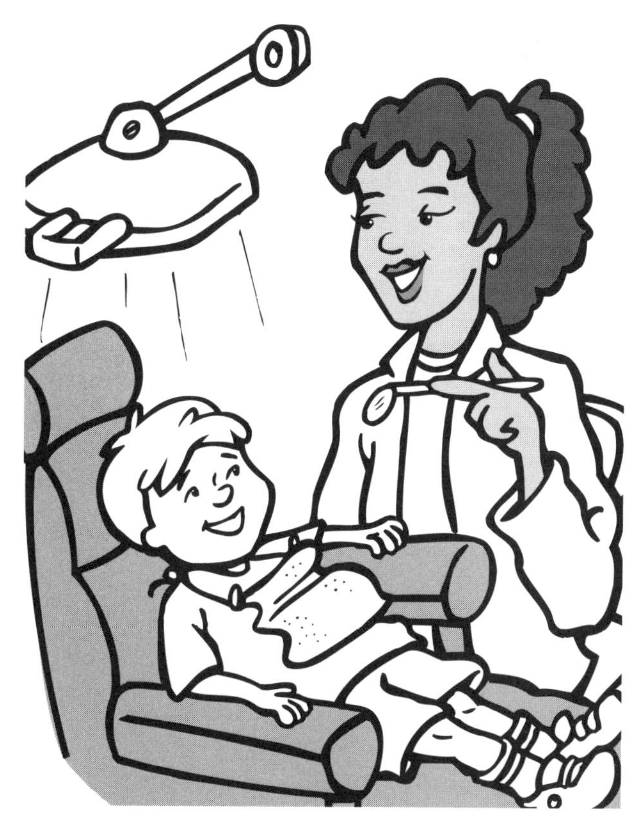

- ***Why*** do people wear a bib at the dentist?

- ***How*** do you take care of your teeth?

1 2 3 4

- ***Who*** is standing near the boy?

- ***Where*** is the little boy?

- ***What*** does a dentist do?

- ***When*** should you visit the dentist?

Cut on dotted line

Doctor's Office

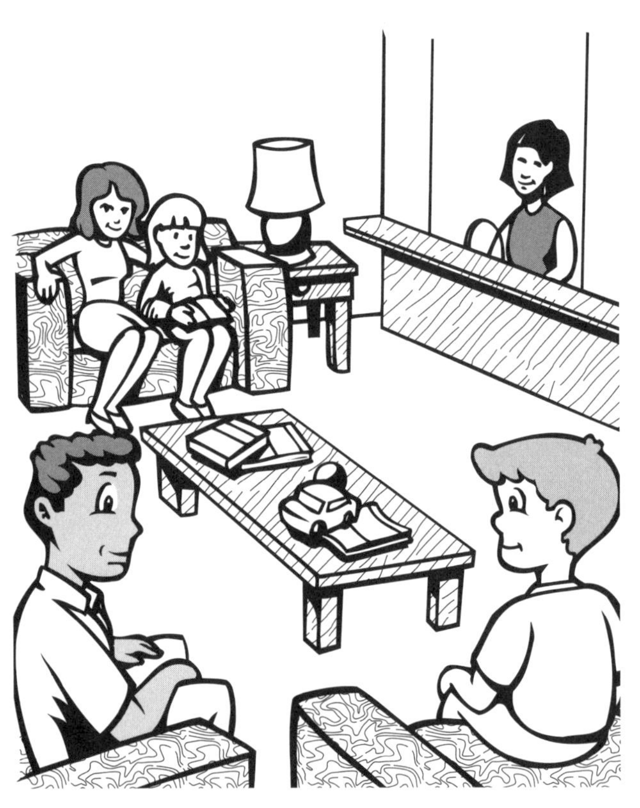

- ***Who*** visits a doctor's office?

- ***What*** do you see in a doctor's office?

- ***Where*** do you wait for the doctor?

- ***When*** do children visit the doctor?

- ***Why*** are books and games in the doctor's office?

- ***How*** do you know when the doctor is ready to see you?

Cut on dotted line

Community

Page 19

Fast Food Restaurant

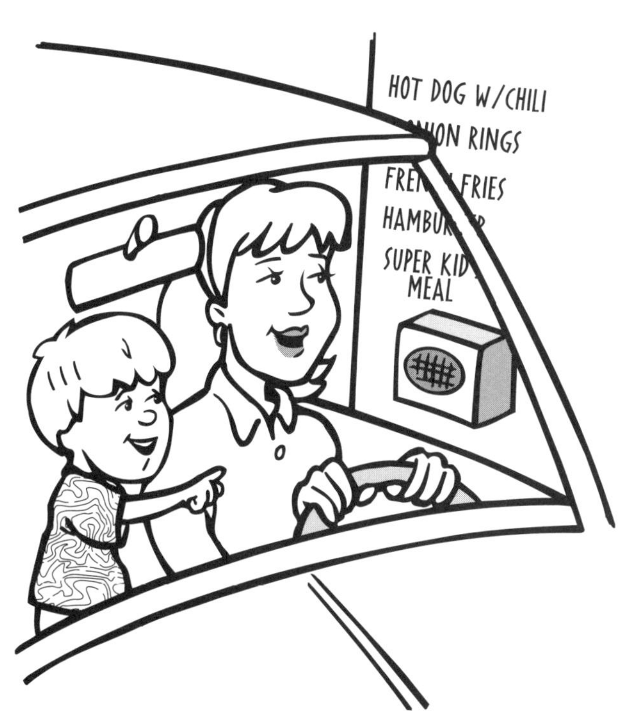

- ***Who*** takes the food order?
- ***What*** will the Mom and her son order?

- ***Where*** is the person who takes the food order?
- ***When*** will Mom pay for the food?

- ***Why*** do some people eat in a restaurant and others use the drive-thru?
- ***How*** will the food taste?

1 2 3 4

Cut on dotted line

Community

Fire Station

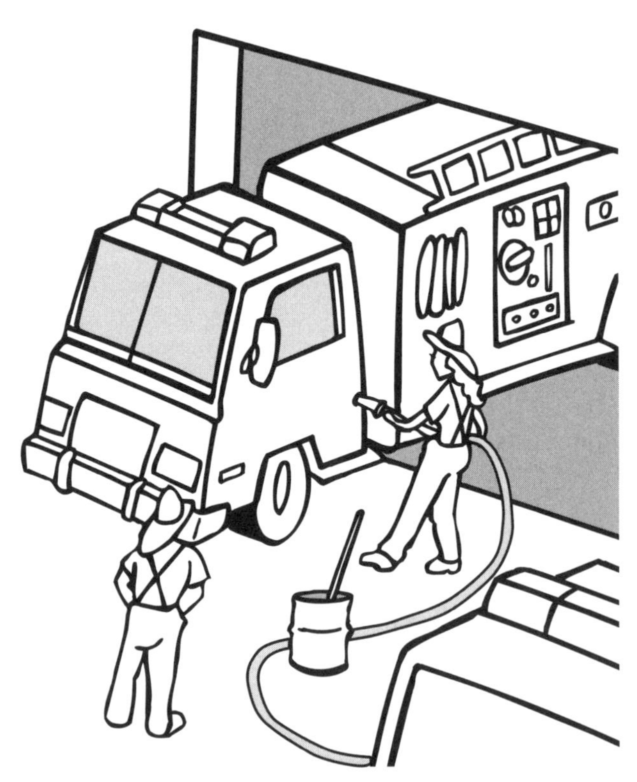

1 2 3 4

- ***Who*** works at the fire station?
- ***What*** type of things are on a fire truck?

- ***Where*** is the fire truck kept?
- ***When*** does a fire truck leave the station?

- ***Why*** do firefighters sleep at the station?
- ***How*** does a person become a firefighter?

Cut on dotted line

Community

Gas Station

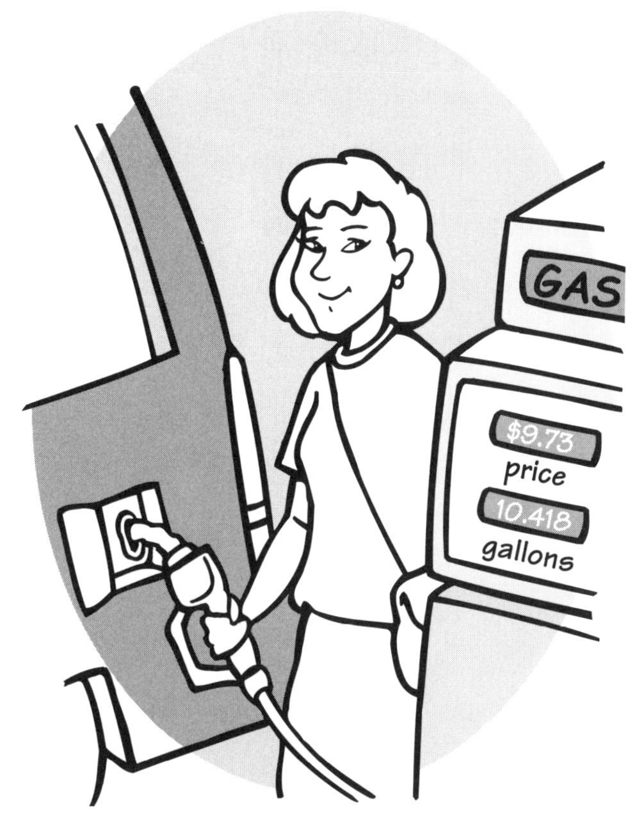

- ***Who*** is using the gas pump?
- ***What*** is the woman doing?

- ***When*** do people go to the gas station?
- ***Where*** will she go after she gets the gas?

- ***Why*** should people not smoke at the gas station?
- ***How*** does the woman know when to stop filling the gas tank?

Grocery Store

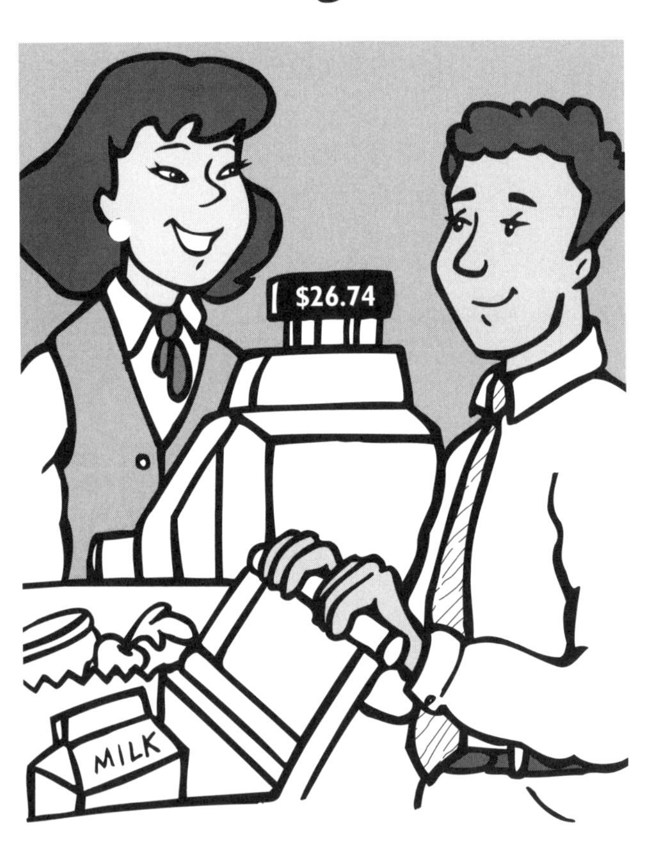

- ***Who*** is using the cash register?
- ***What*** is the man pushing?

- ***Where*** is the man?
- ***When*** will he be finished shopping?

- ***Why*** did the man go shopping?
- ***How*** will he get the food to his car?

1 2 3 4

Cut on dotted line

Community

Cut on dotted line

Ice Cream Shop

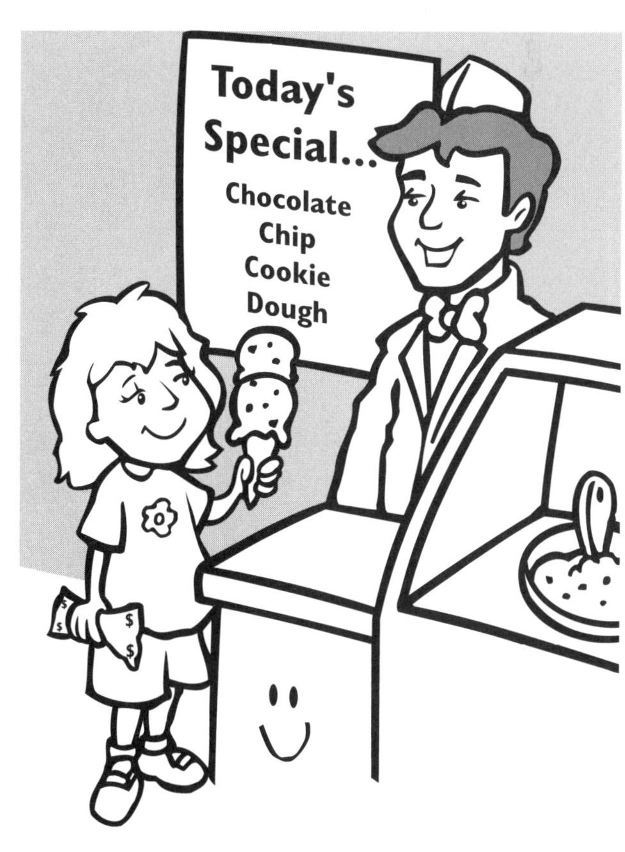

1 2 3 4

- ***Who*** is buying an ice cream cone?
- ***What*** does the worker use to put the ice cream into the cone?
- ***Where*** can people buy ice cream?
- ***When*** is the best time to eat ice cream?
- ***Why*** does the girl have money in her hand?
- ***How*** often do you eat ice cream?

Juice Machine

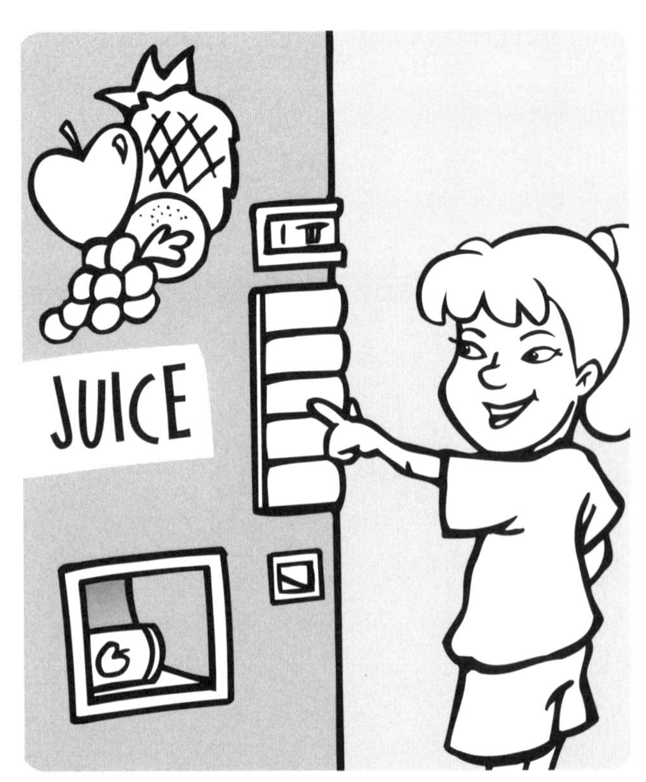

- ***Who*** is getting some juice?
- ***What*** type of juice did the girl get?
- ***Where*** is the girl?
- ***When*** can the girl get some more juice?
- ***Why*** is the girl getting her juice?
- ***How*** does the machine work?

1 2 3 4

Cut on dotted line

Cut on dotted line

- ***What*** is the girl doing?

- ***When*** did the girl write the letter?

- ***Who*** works at a post office?

- ***Where*** will the letter be sent?

2 3
1 4

Post Office

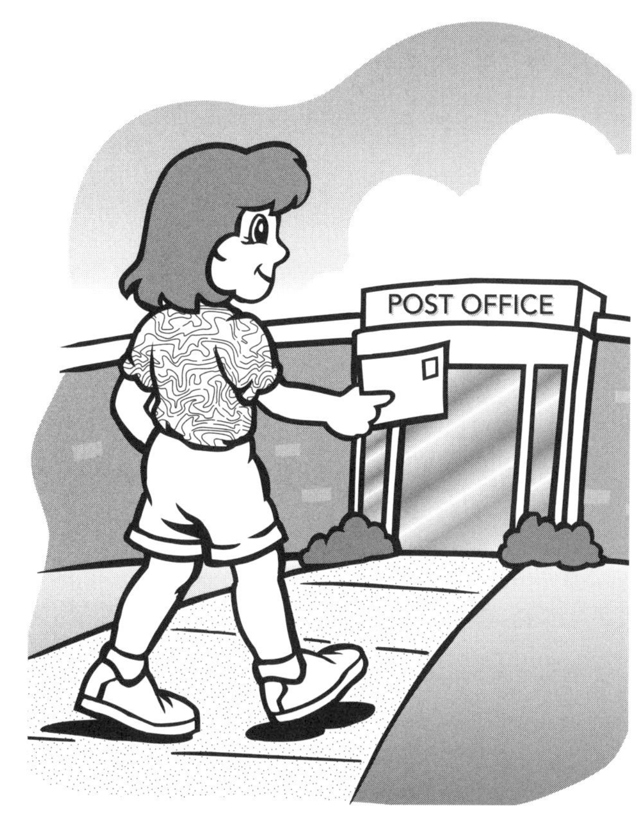

- ***Why*** do people send letters?

- ***How*** do you get to your post office?

Movie Ticket Line

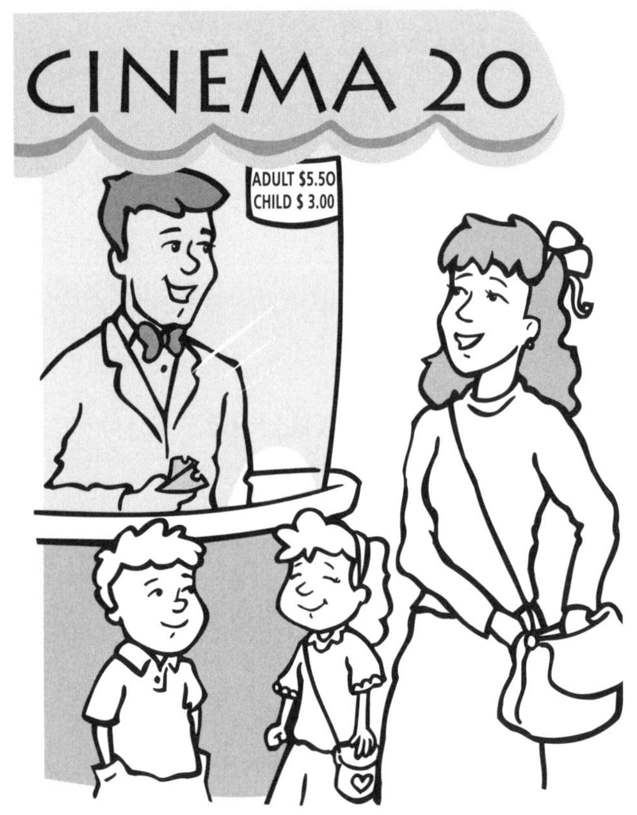

- ***Who*** is buying the movie tickets?
- ***What*** do people eat at the movies?

- ***Where*** is the man who sells the tickets?
- ***When*** do people go to the movies?

- ***Why*** do people need tickets to get into a movie?
- ***How*** many tickets does the woman need?

Cut on dotted line

- ***What*** do you call people who break the law?

- ***When*** do policemen work?

- ***Who*** is inside the police car?

- ***Where*** is the police car going?

2 3
1 4

Police Car

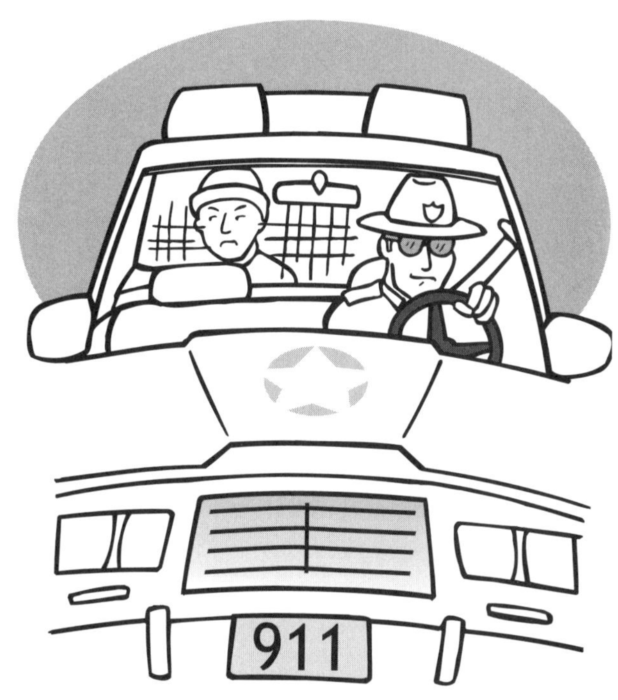

- ***Why*** do we need the police?

- ***How*** do police officers help people?

Cut on dotted line

Restaurant

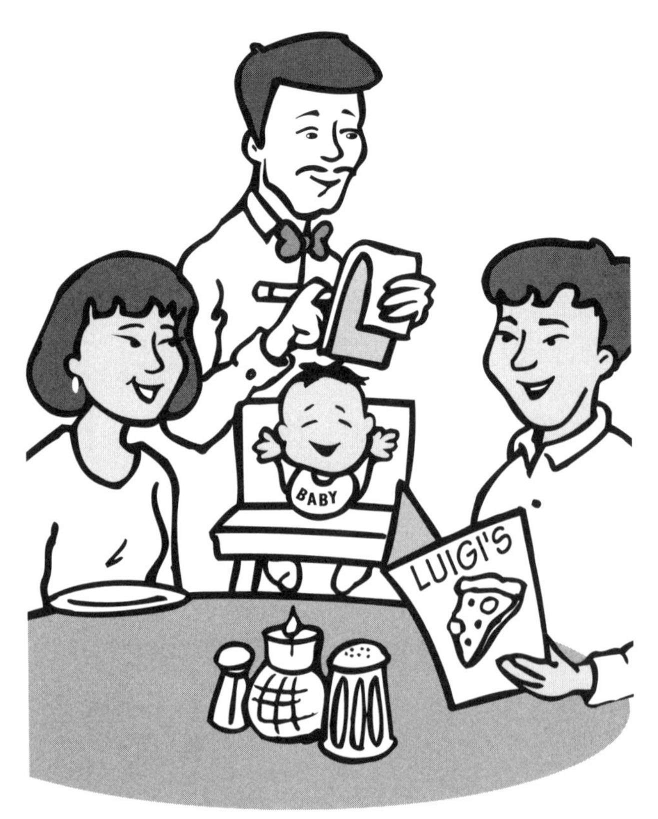

- ***Who*** is taking the food order?
- ***What*** is the Dad reading?
- ***Where*** is the baby sitting?
- ***When*** do people eat at a restaurant?
- ***Why*** is the person writing down the order?
- ***How*** does the waiter carry the food order?

Cut on dotted line

Vet

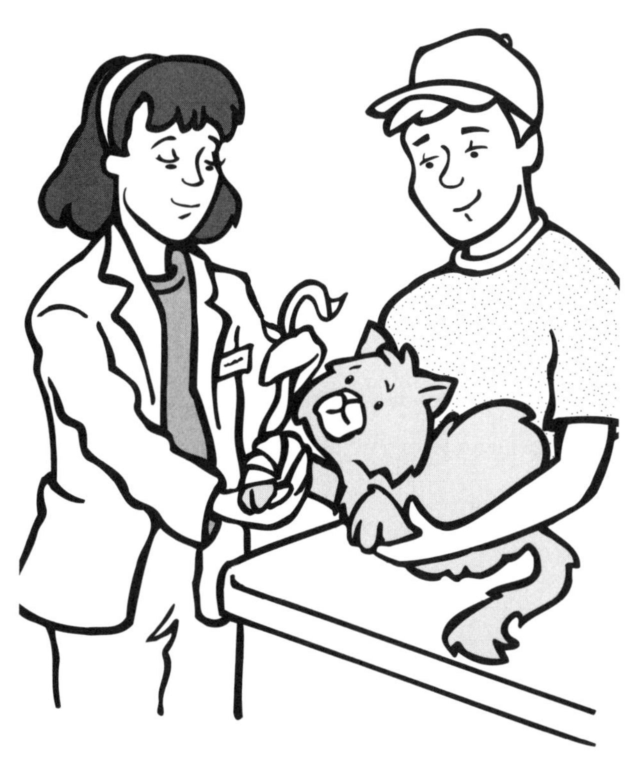

1 2 3 4

- ***Who*** takes care of sick animals?
- ***What*** is the woman doing?

- ***Where*** is the cat?
- ***When*** will the bandage be removed?

- ***Why*** is the man holding the cat?
- ***How*** did the cat hurt its paw?

Zoo

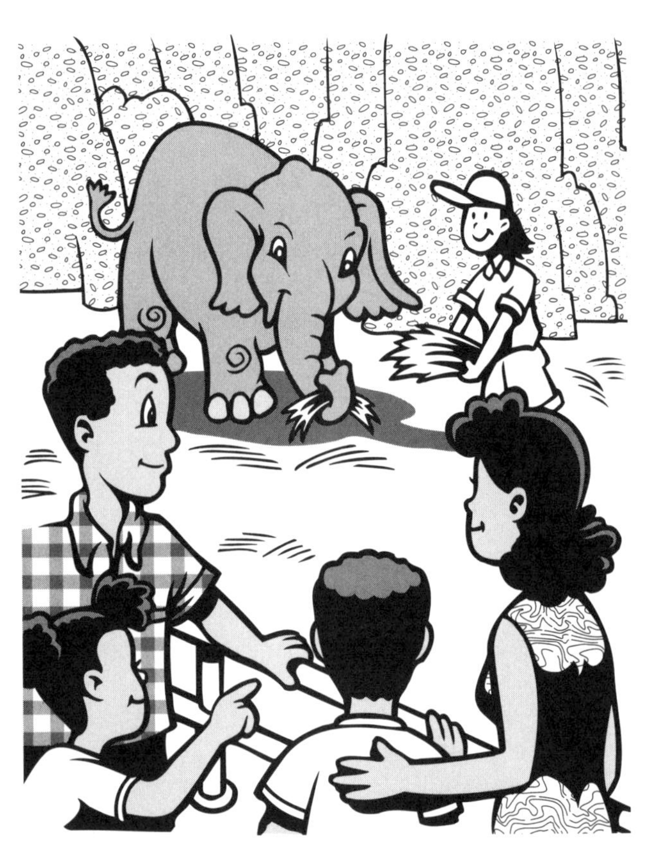

- ***Who*** is feeding the elephant?
- ***What*** do elephants like to eat?
- ***Where*** is the family?
- ***When*** do animals sleep?
- ***Why*** are the animals in cages?
- ***How*** do you feed an elephant?

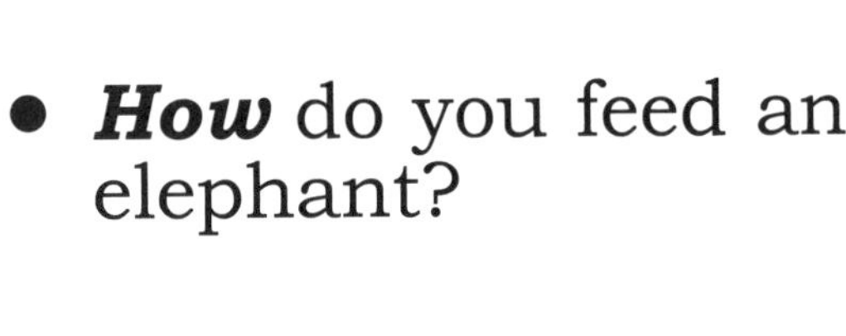

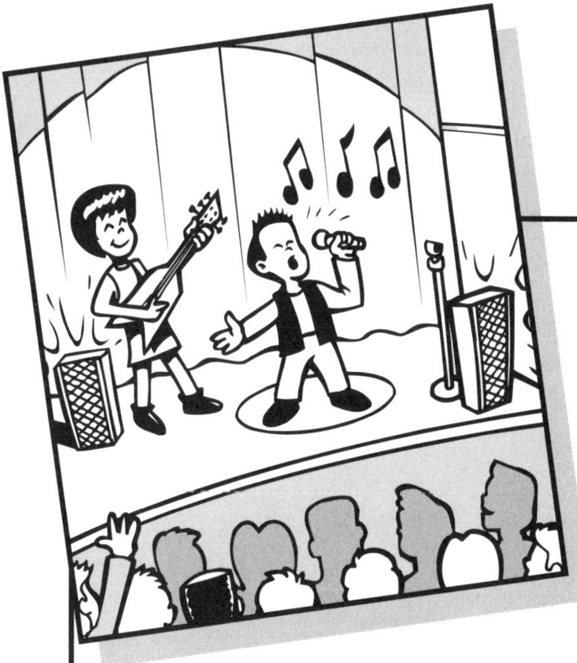

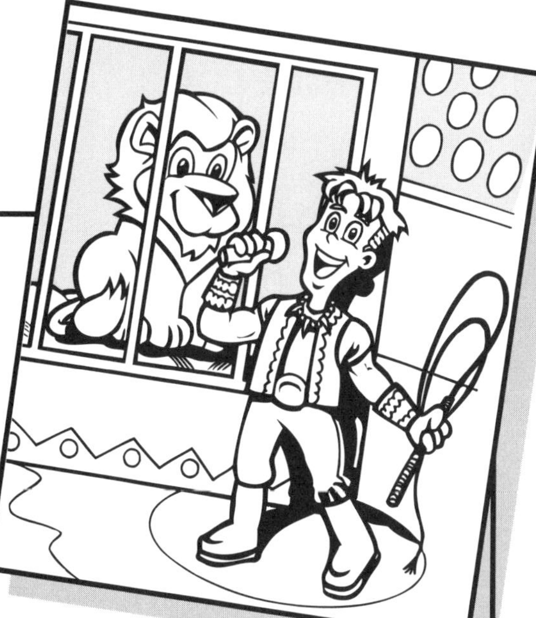

Entertainment

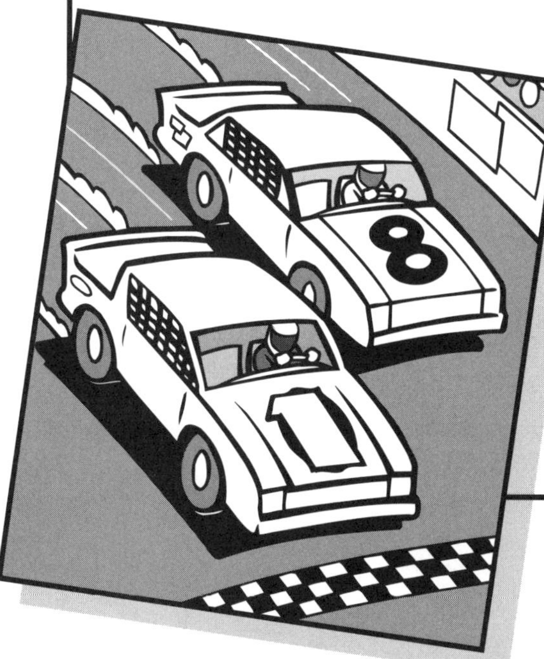

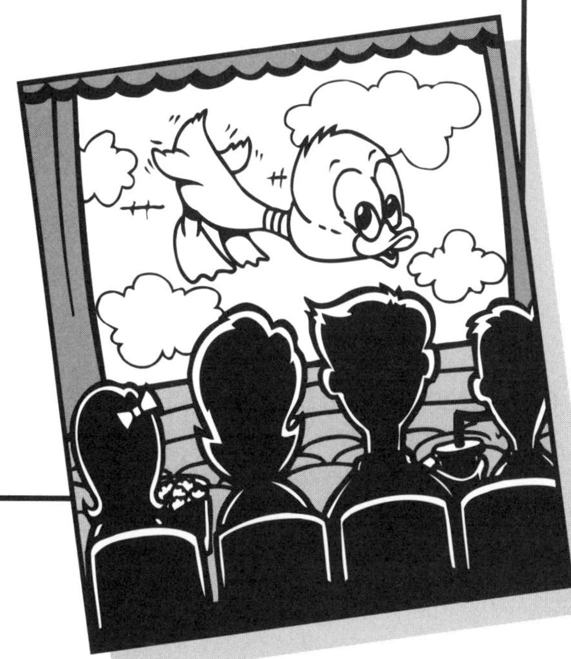

Ballet

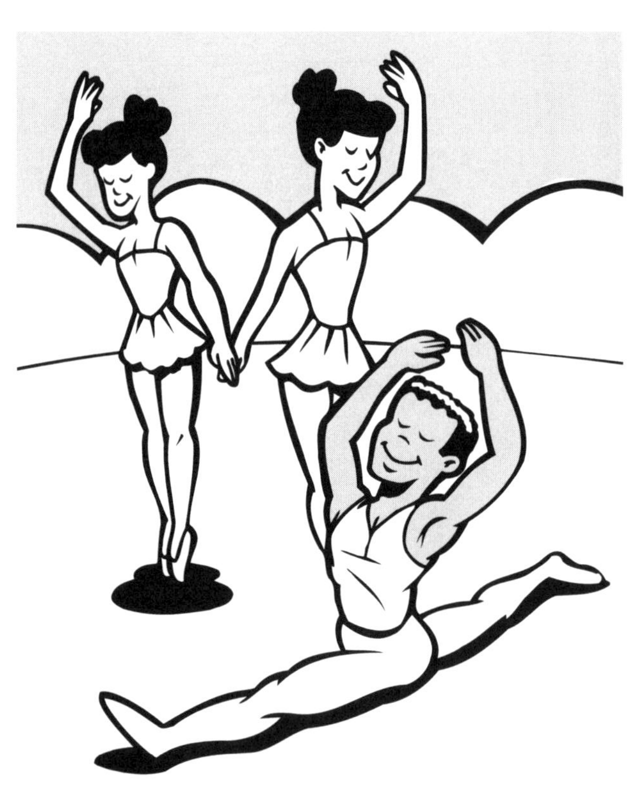

- ***Who*** is dancing on their tiptoes?
- ***What*** is the boy doing?
- ***Where*** is the boy?
- ***When*** do ballet dancers practice?
- ***Why*** do dancers wear special shoes?
- ***How*** do ballet dancers dance?

1 2 3 4

Cut on dotted line

Entertainment

Cut on dotted line

Entertainment

Circus

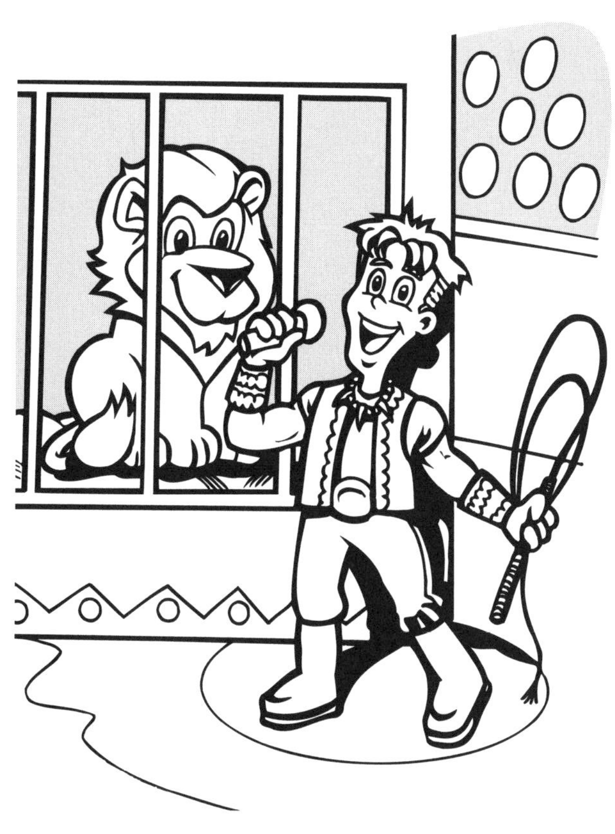

- ***Who*** has the microphone?
- ***What*** animals do you see at the circus?

- ***Where*** is the lion?
- ***When*** do people go to the circus?

- ***Why*** does the man need a microphone?
- ***How*** does the circus get to your town?

1 2 3 4

Cut on dotted line

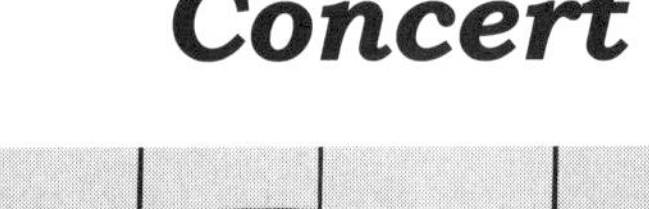

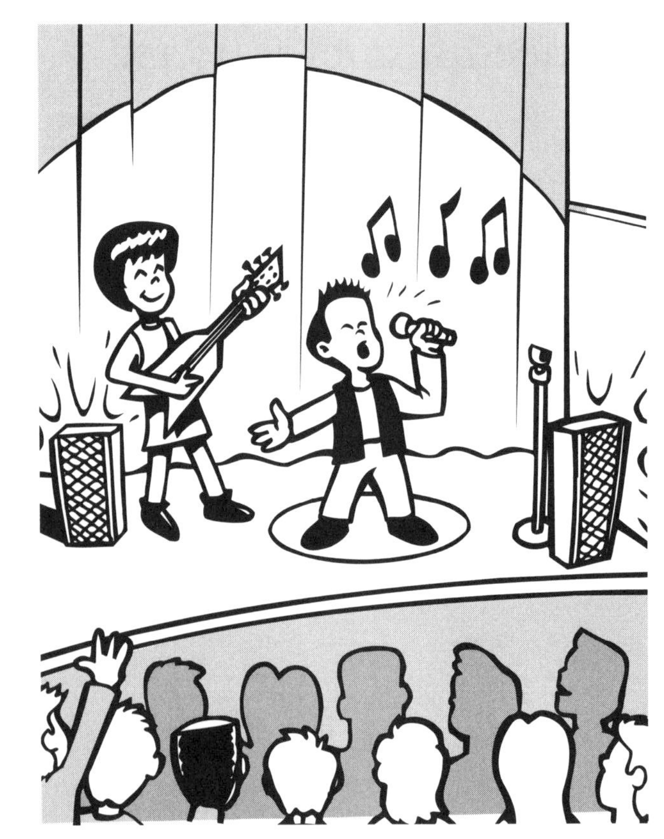

1 2 3 4

- ***Who*** is singing?
- ***What*** is the woman playing?
- ***Where*** are the boy and woman?
- ***When*** does a performer hold the microphone up to his mouth?
- ***Why*** are concerts on stage?
- ***How*** is a guitar played?

Cut on dotted line

Entertainment

Fair

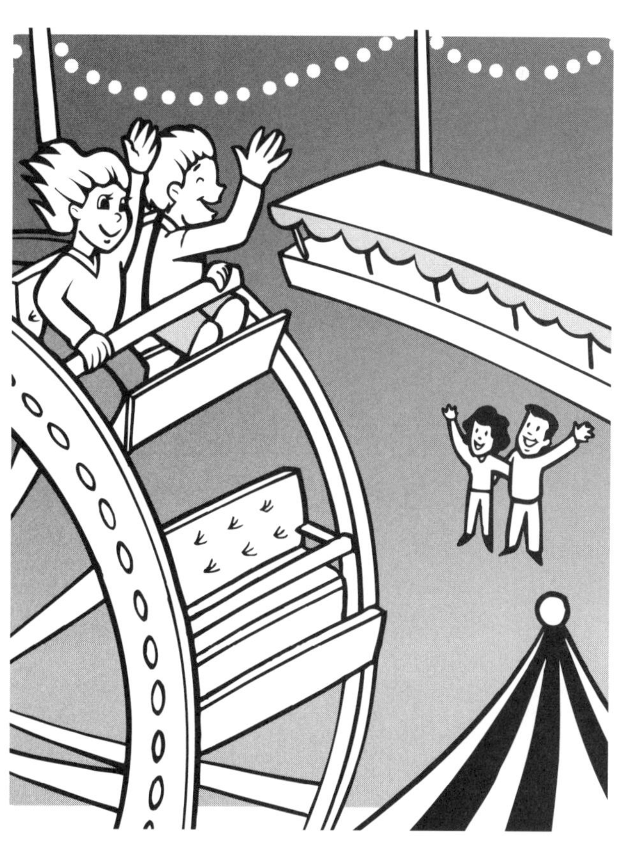

- ***Who*** is on the ride?

- ***What*** are they sitting in?

- ***Where*** are their parents?

- ***When*** will they get off the ride?

1 2 3 4

- ***Why*** is there a bar across their laps?

- ***How*** did they get into the seat?

Movie Theater

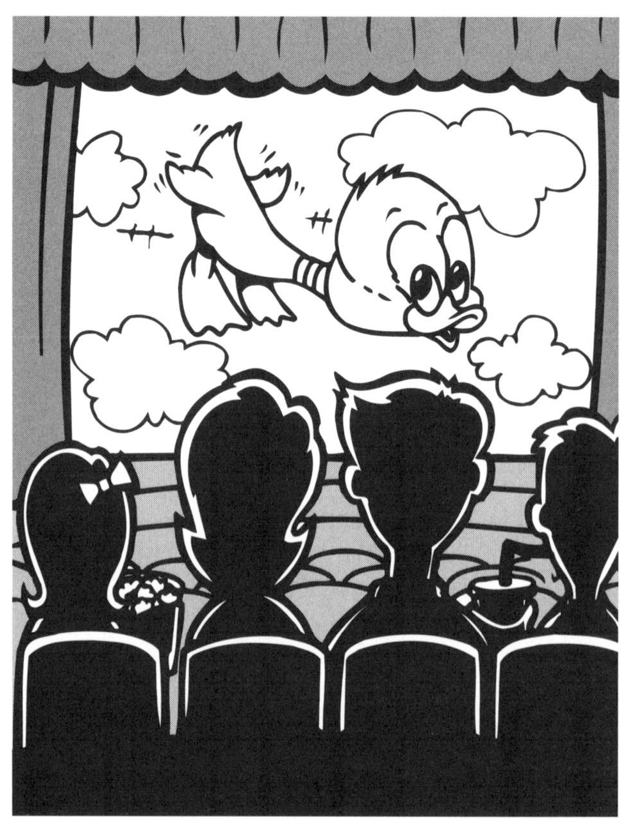

- ***Who*** is sitting beside the Father?
- ***What*** is this family watching?

- ***Where*** is the movie screen?
- ***When*** do people leave their seats at the movies?

- ***Why*** do people go to the movies?
- ***How*** do people behave at the movies?

1 2 3 4

Cut on dotted line

Cut on dotted line

Entertainment

Orchestra

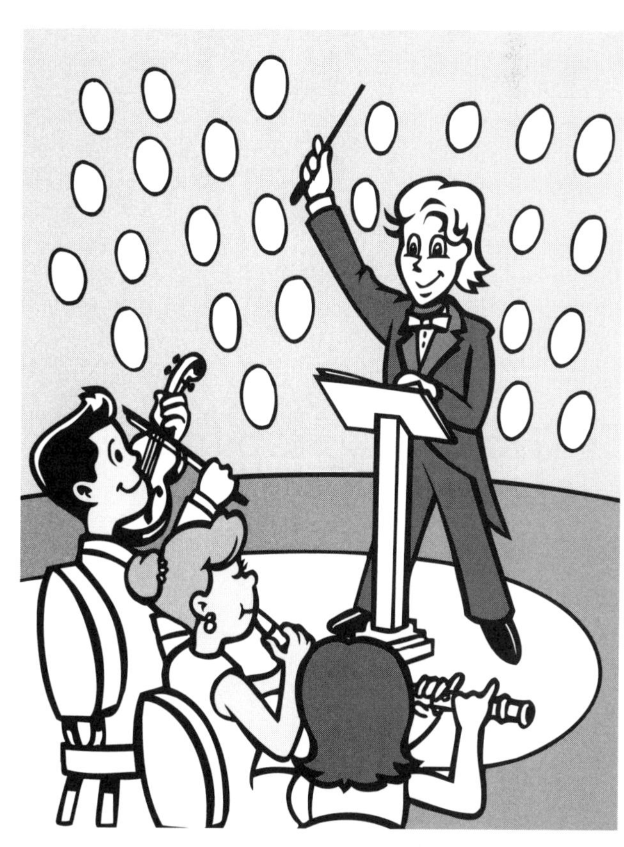

2 3

1 4

- ***Who*** leads the orchestra?
- ***What*** are these musicians playing?
- ***Where*** does the conductor stand?
- ***When*** does an audience clap?
- ***Why*** does an audience go to hear an orchestra?
- ***How*** do musicians know when to play their instruments?

Cut on dotted line

Entertainment

Parade

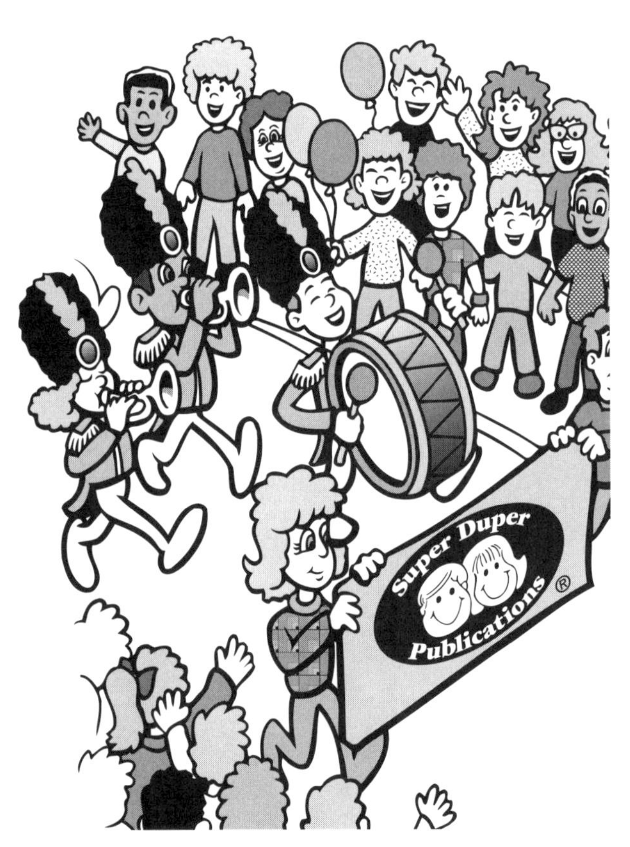

- ***Who*** is playing the drum?
- ***What*** are the children in the front carrying?

- ***Where*** is the marching band?
- ***When*** might you see a parade?

- ***Why*** do people have parades?
- ***How*** does a band walk in a parade?

Cut on dotted line

Play

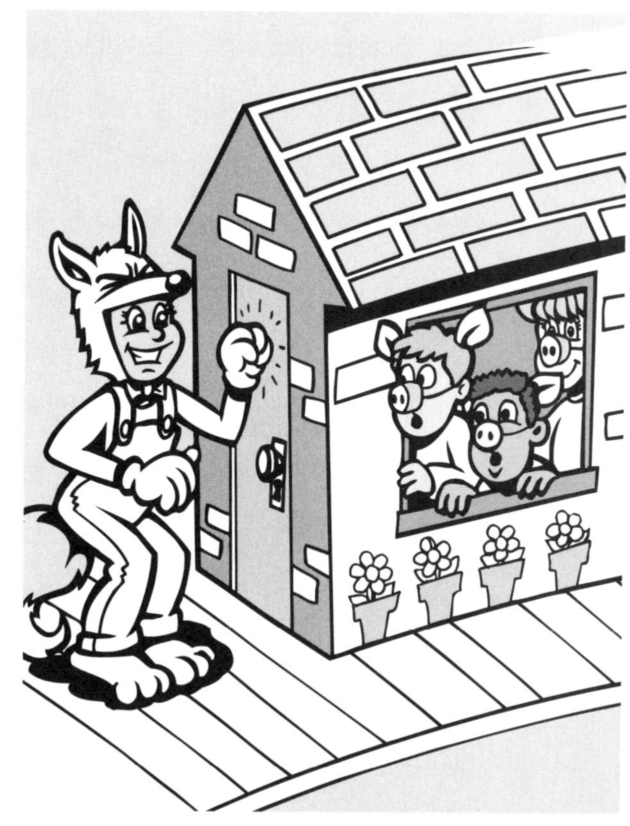

1 2 3 4

- ***What*** was used to make this house?
- ***Who*** is knocking on the door at the house?

- ***When*** do people wear costumes?
- ***Where*** are the little boys?

- ***Why*** do people knock on doors?
- ***How*** do the pigs feel?

Cut on dotted line

Racetrack

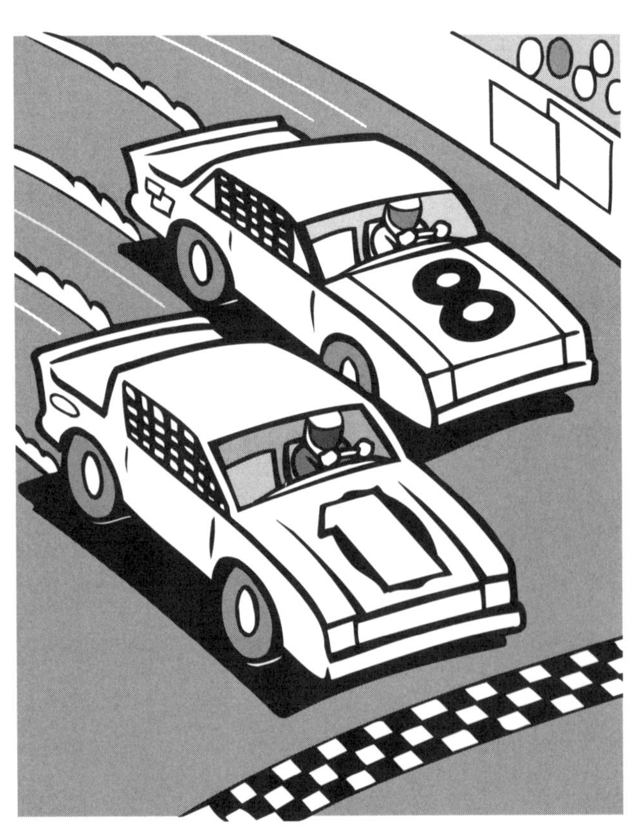

- ***Who*** drives a car like this?
- ***What*** is on the driver's head?

- ***Where*** is the winner?
- ***When*** is the race over?

- ***Why*** do people race?
- ***How*** do racers drive?

Rodeo

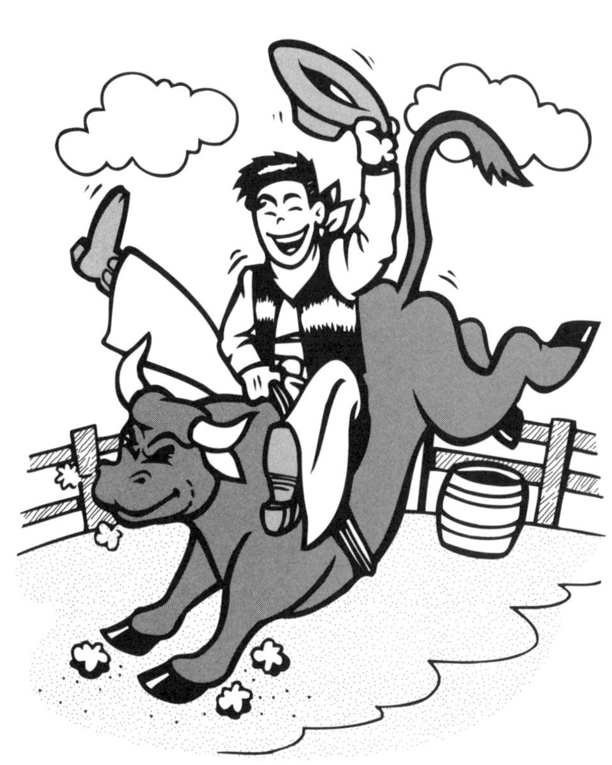

- ***Who*** is riding the bull?
- ***What*** is the cowboy wearing?
- ***Where*** does a cowboy ride a bull?
- ***When*** does a cowboy get up in the morning?
- ***Why*** is the bull trying to throw the cowboy to the ground?
- ***How*** does the cowboy hang on?

Cut on dotted line

Sports Event/Stadium

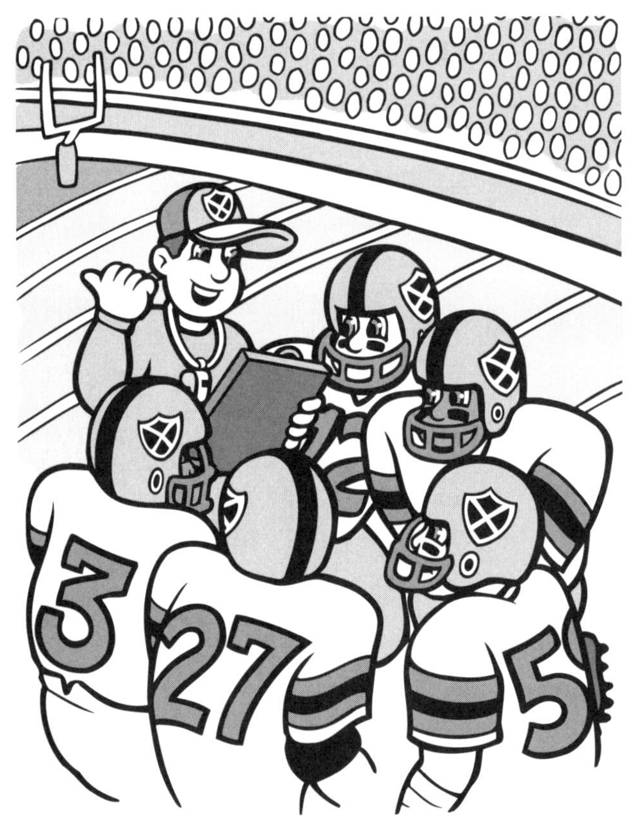

1 2 3 4

- ***Who*** is talking to the players?
- ***What*** are the players wearing on their heads?

- ***Where*** are the players?
- ***When*** does a coach talk to his players?

- ***Why*** do football players wear helmets and pads?
- ***How*** do people get to a sports stadium?

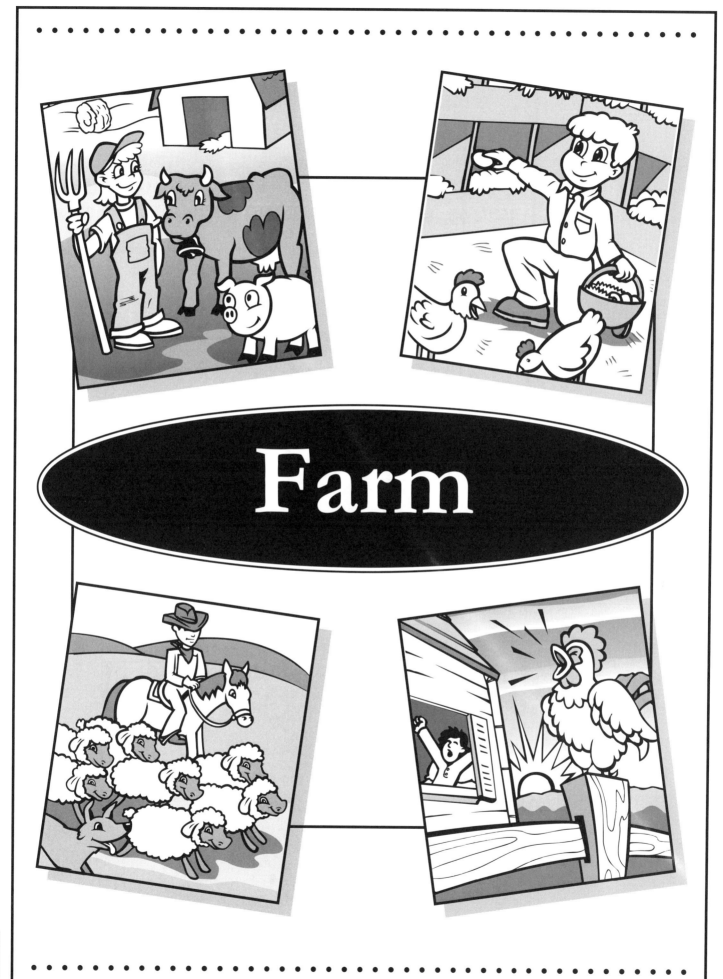

Farm

Cut on dotted line

Collecting Eggs

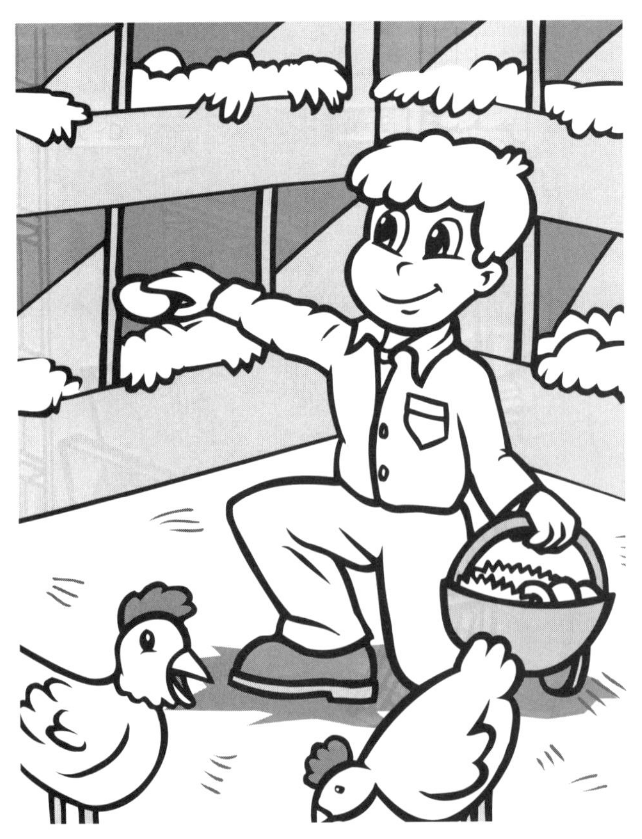

- ***Who*** is collecting the eggs?
- ***What*** does he put the eggs in?

- ***Where*** are the chickens?
- ***When*** do you eat eggs?

- ***Why*** do you have to be careful with eggs?
- ***How*** do you make sure the eggs don't break?

Cut on dotted line

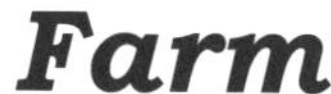

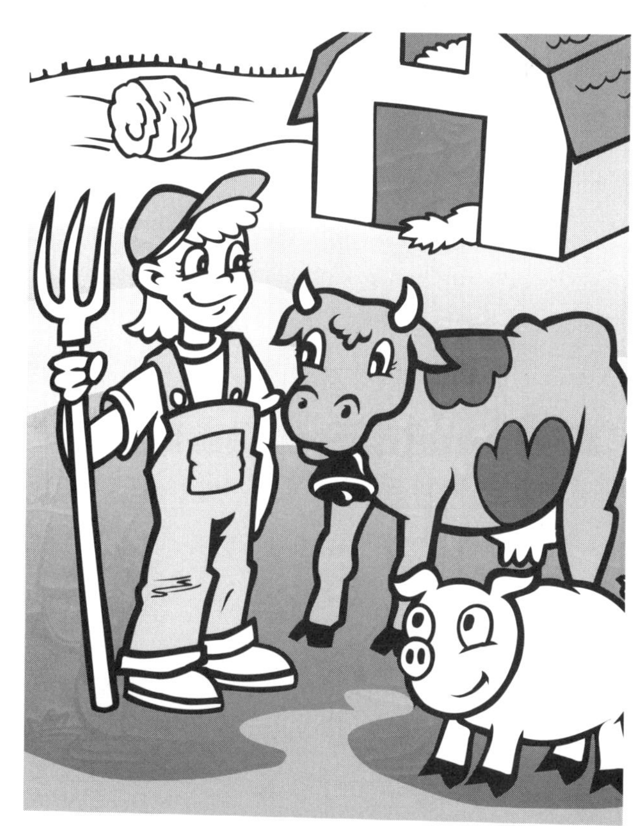

1 2 3 4

- ***Who*** feeds the animals?

- ***What*** is the cow wearing?

- ***Where*** do a pig and a cow live?

- ***When*** do animals go into the barn?

- ***Why*** does the barn have straw?

- ***How*** do animals stay warm?

Cut on dotted line

Farm

Feeding Animals

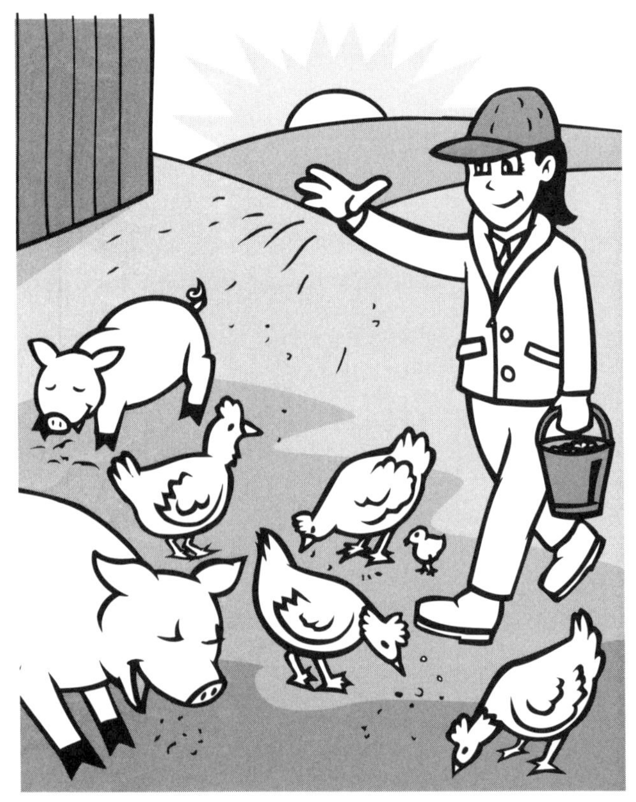

1 2 3 4

- ***Who*** is feeding the animals?
- ***What*** does she keep the animal feed in?

- ***Where*** does she keep the pigs?
- ***When*** is she feeding the animals?

- ***Why*** do the animals look so happy?
- ***How*** do you feed a pig?

Cut on dotted line

- ***What*** are they doing?

- ***When*** do you go on a hayride?

- ***Who*** is on the hayride?

- ***Where*** are they going?

1 2 3 4

Hayride

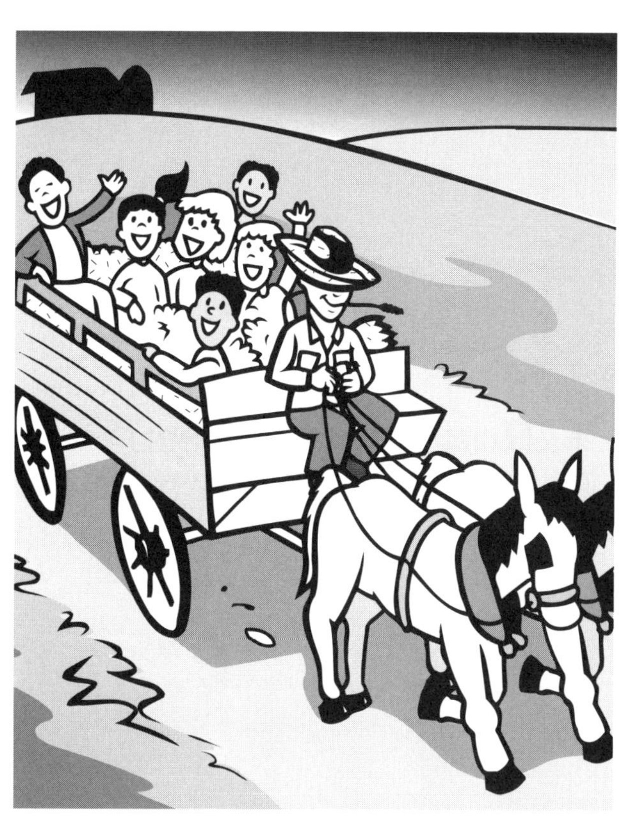

- ***Why*** are they singing?

- ***How*** do the horses know where to go?

Herding Sheep

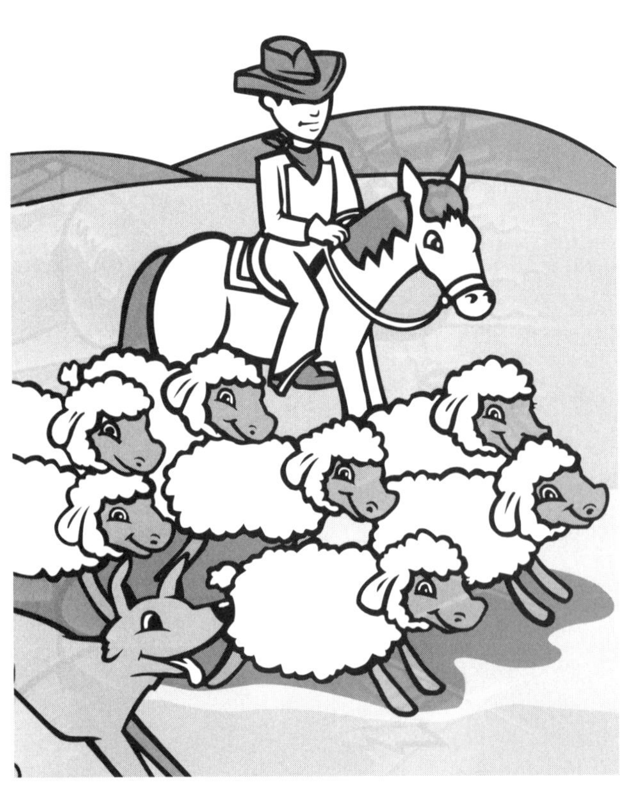

- ***Who*** keeps the sheep all together?
- ***What*** is he riding on?

- ***Where*** do sheep live?
- ***When*** do the sheep escape?

- ***Why*** is the cowboy on a horse?
- ***How*** does a sheepdog keep the sheep together?

Cut on dotted line

Cut on dotted line

Farm

2 3
1 4

Horseshoeing

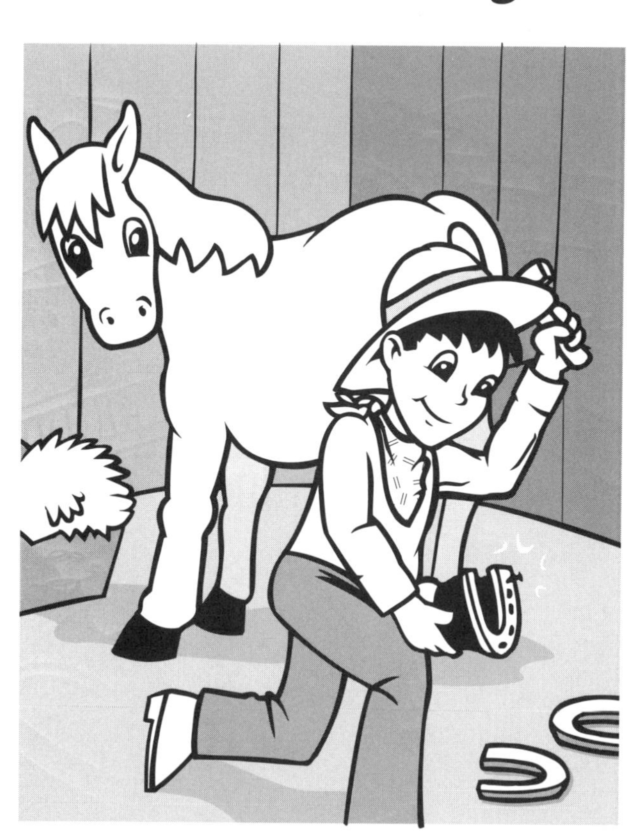

- ***Who*** is putting shoes on the horse?
- ***What*** is on his head?

- ***Where*** do the horseshoes go?
- ***When*** does a horse wear shoes?

- ***Why*** does a horse wear shoes?
- ***How*** do you know if a horse needs new shoes?

Milking a Cow

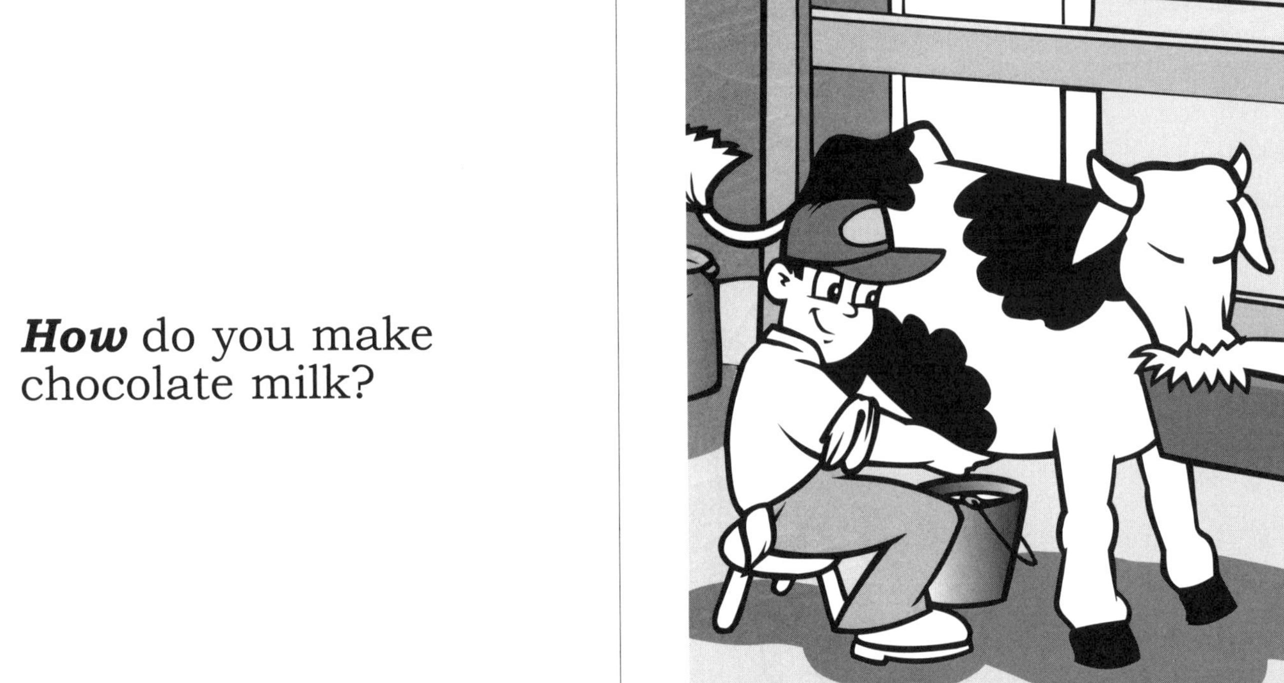

- ***Who*** is milking the cow?
- ***What*** does the cow make?
- ***Where*** is the stool?
- ***When*** do you drink milk?
- ***Why*** do we drink milk?
- ***How*** do you make chocolate milk?

1 2 3 4

Cut on dotted line

- ***What*** is the rooster sitting on?
- ***Who*** hears the rooster?

- ***When*** does a rooster crow?
- ***Where*** is the farmer?

2 3
1 4

Rooster

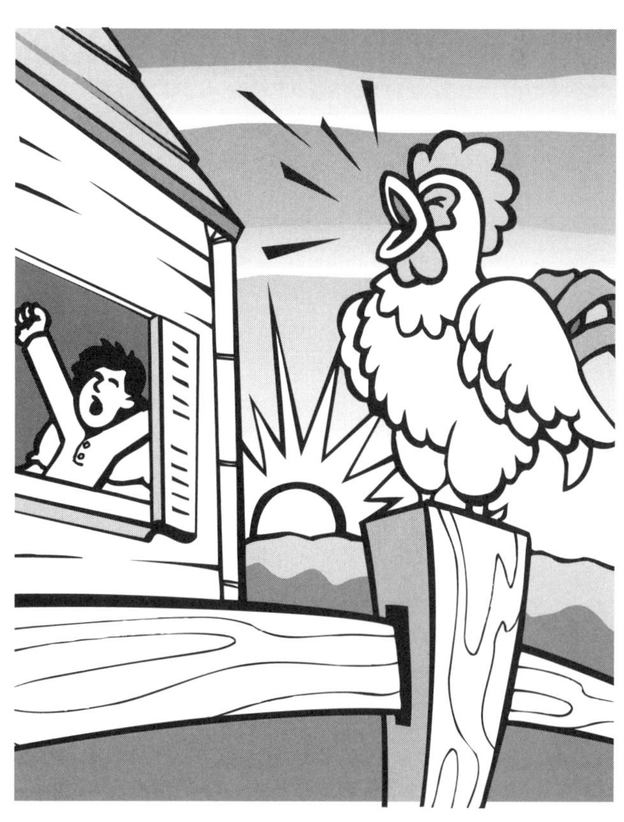

- ***Why*** is the farmer awake?

- ***How*** do you wake up in the morning?

Cut on dotted line

Farm

Tractor

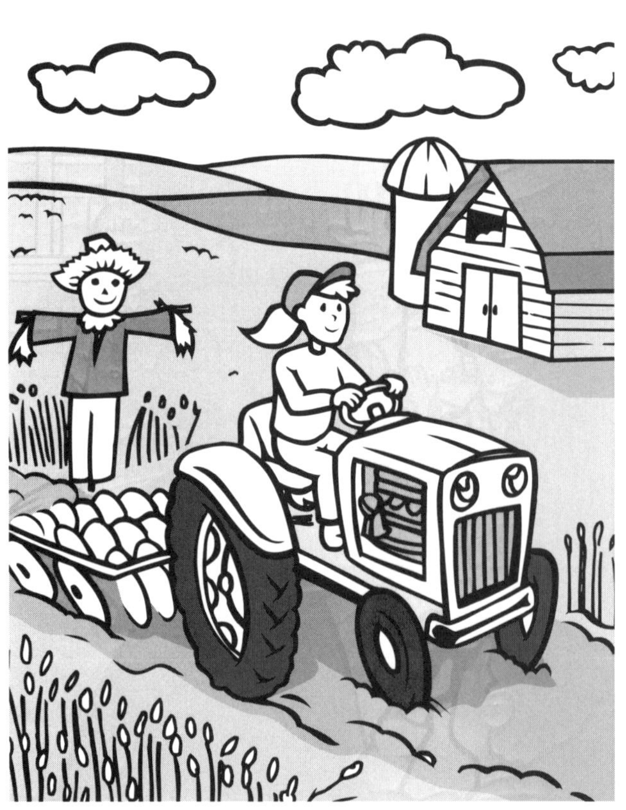

1 2 3 4

- ***Who*** is riding the tractor?
- ***What*** else is in the field?

- ***Where*** is the farmer sitting?
- ***When*** does a farmer plow her field?

- ***Why*** is there a scarecrow in the field?
- ***How*** do you make a scarecrow?

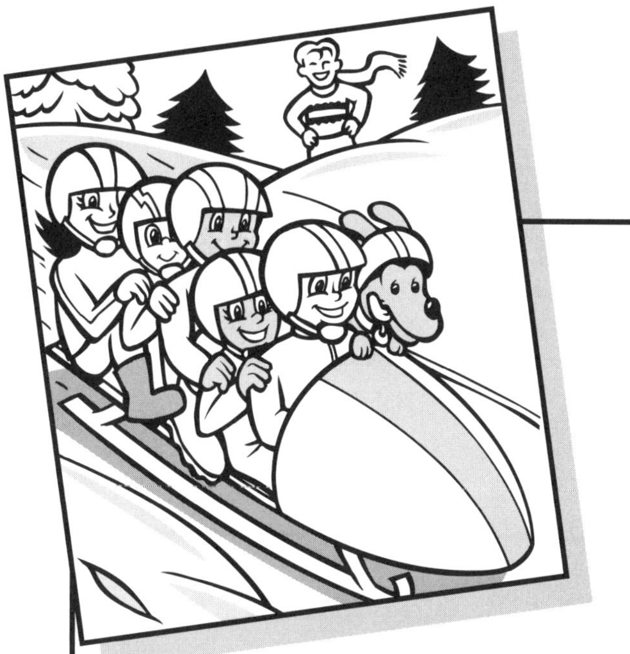

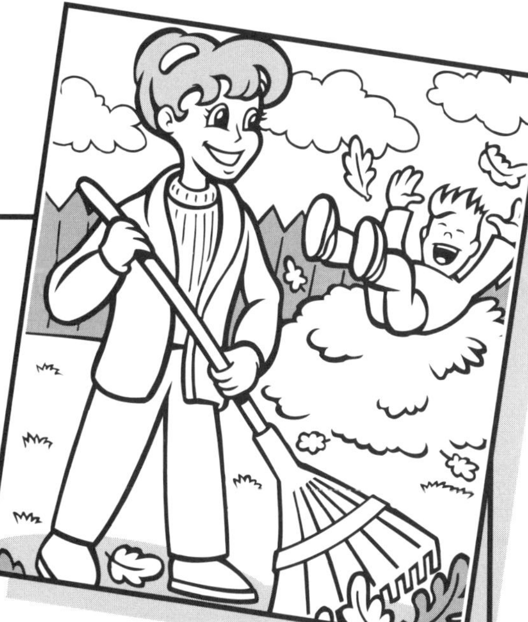

Holiday, Seasonal & Special Occasions

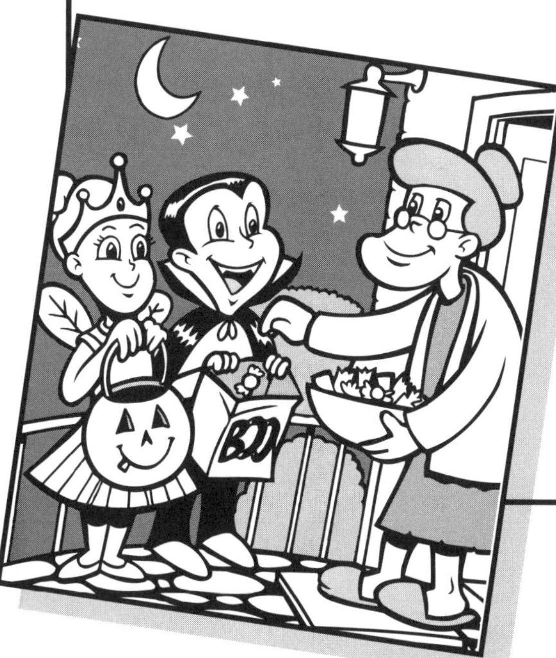

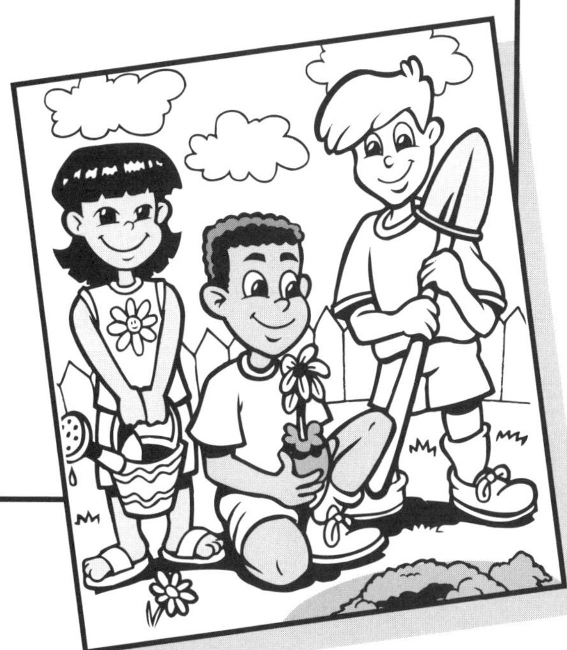

Birthday Party

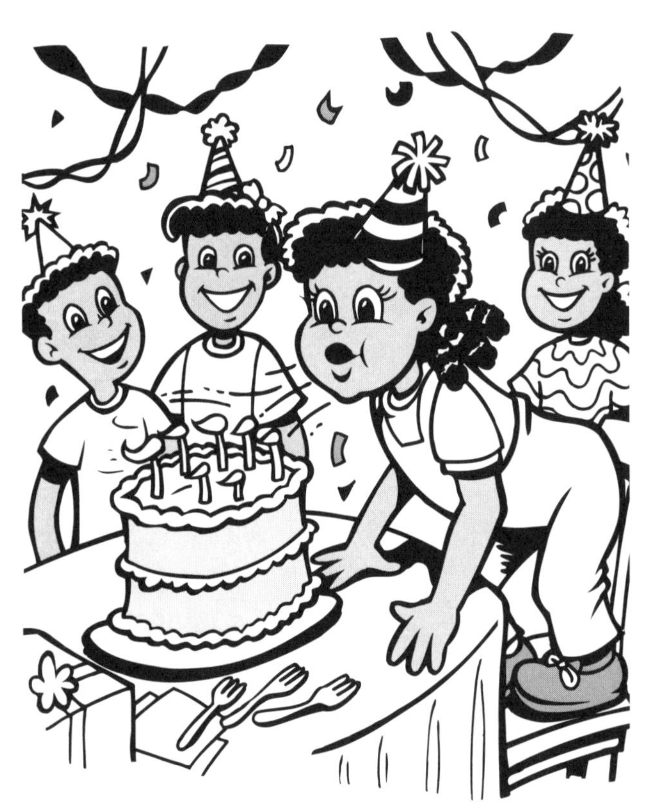

- ***Who*** is blowing out the candles?
- ***What*** are the children wearing on their heads?

- ***Where*** are the candles?
- ***When*** does the birthday person make a wish?

- ***Why*** do people celebrate birthdays?
- ***How*** do you feel at a party?

1 2 3 4

Cut on dotted line

Christmas Tree

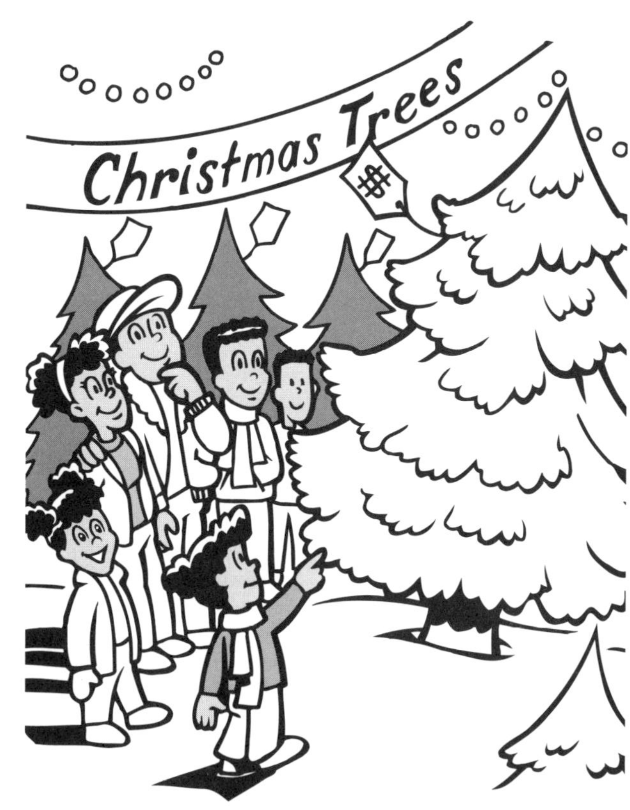

1 2 3 4

- ***Who*** is pointing at the tree?
- ***What*** is on the tree?
- ***Where*** do families buy trees?
- ***When*** do people decorate trees?
- ***Why*** does this family like this tree?
- ***How*** will the family take this tree home?

Cut on dotted line

Cut on dotted line

- ***When*** will the children eat the eggs?

- ***Where*** can you find an egg?

- ***What*** are the children carrying?

- ***Who*** hid these eggs?

3 2
4 1

Easter Egg Hunt

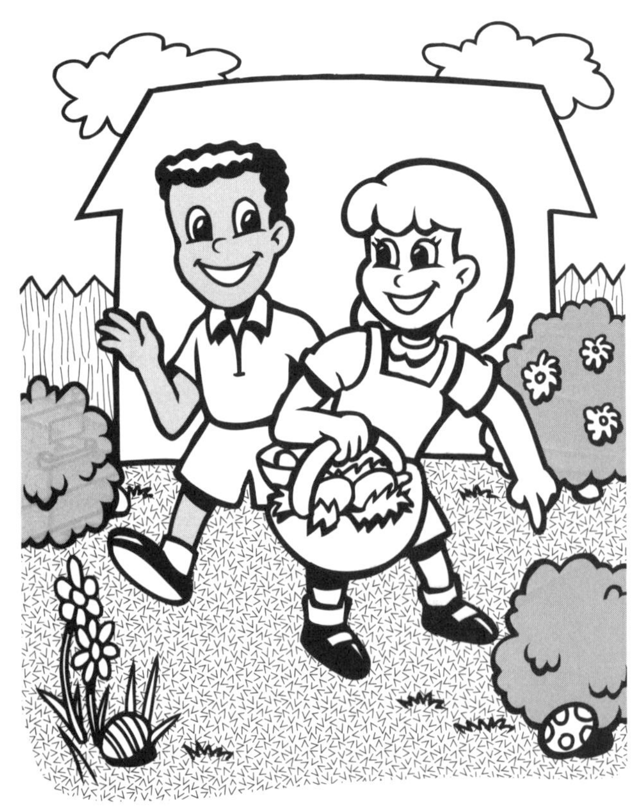

- ***Why*** are the children carrying baskets?

- ***How*** do people color eggs?

Cut on dotted line

Father's Day

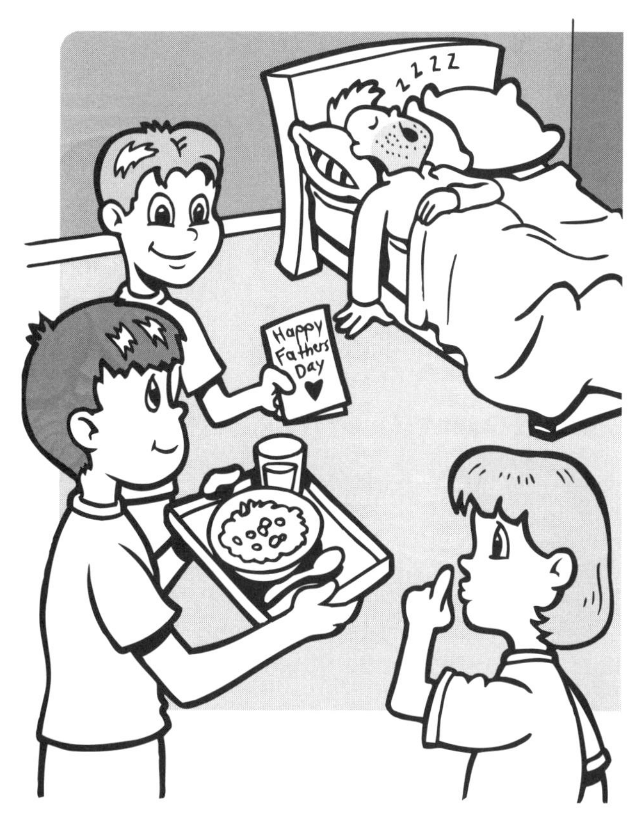

1 2 3 4

- ***Who*** is sleeping?
- ***What*** is on the tray?

- ***Where*** will this father eat his breakfast?
- ***When*** does a dad go to work?

- ***Why*** did these children bring their father breakfast?
- ***How*** will this father feel when he wakes up?

Flag Day

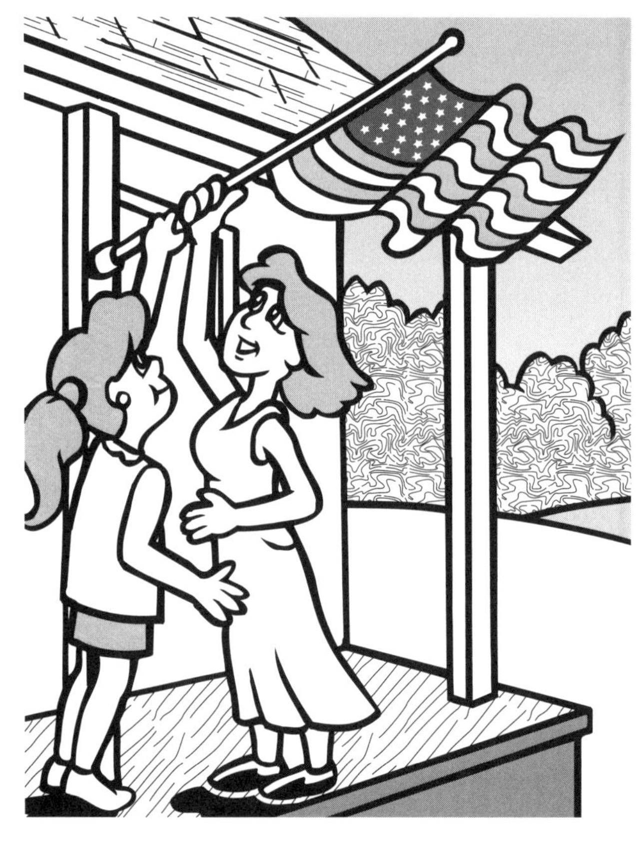

- ***Who*** is on the porch?
- ***What*** are they putting out?

- ***Where*** is the flag holder?
- ***When*** do we put out flags?

- ***Why*** do countries have different flags?
- ***How*** do you make a flag?

1 2 3 4

Cut on dotted line

4th of July

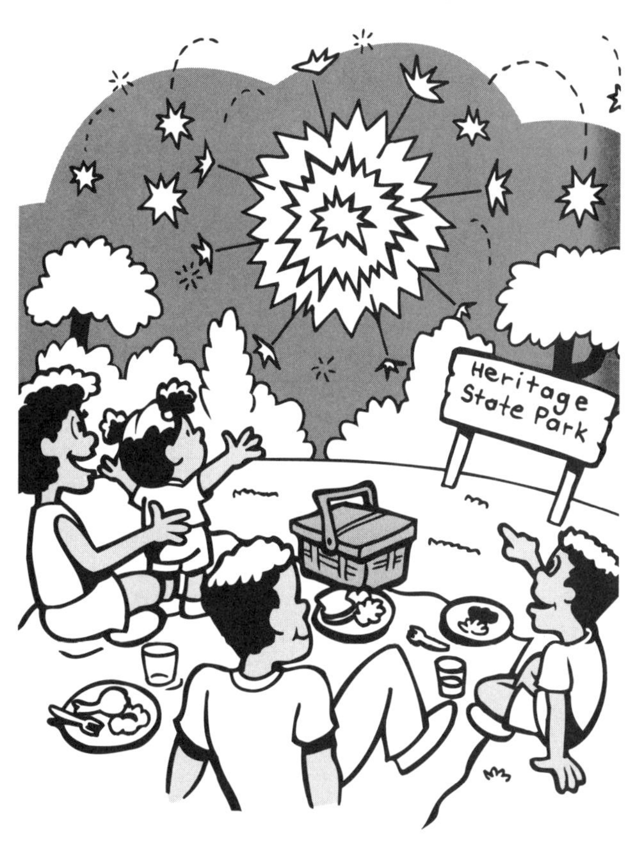

1 2
4 3

- ***Who*** is watching fireworks?
- ***What*** is in the sky?

- ***Where*** are these people eating?
- ***When*** do you see fireworks?

- ***Why*** do people in the USA celebrate the 4th of July?
- ***How*** do Americans celebrate the 4th of July?

Graduation

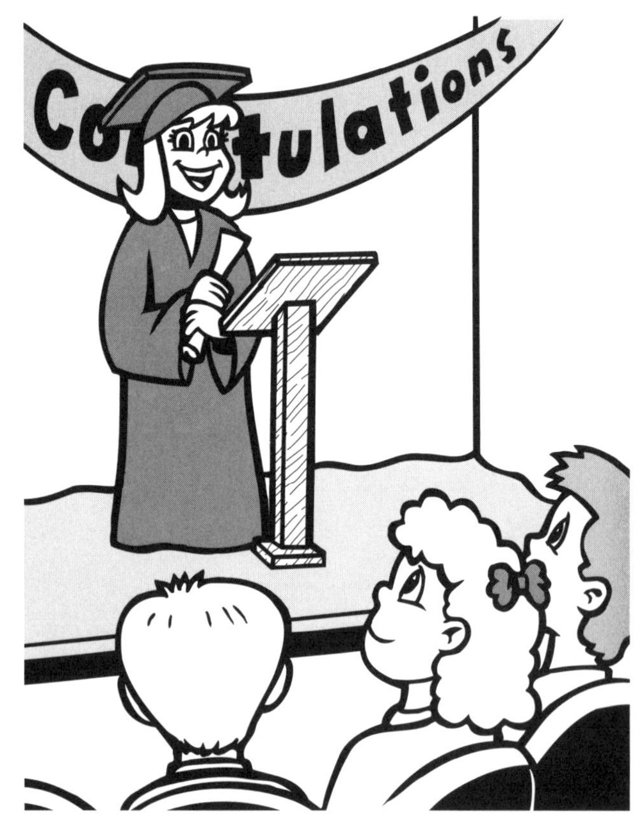

- ***Who*** is graduating?
- ***What*** is the graduate holding?
- ***Where*** should a student stand to give a speech?
- ***When*** do students graduate?
- ***Why*** is graduation special?
- ***How*** do graduating students dress?

Cut on dotted line

Cut on dotted line

Halloween

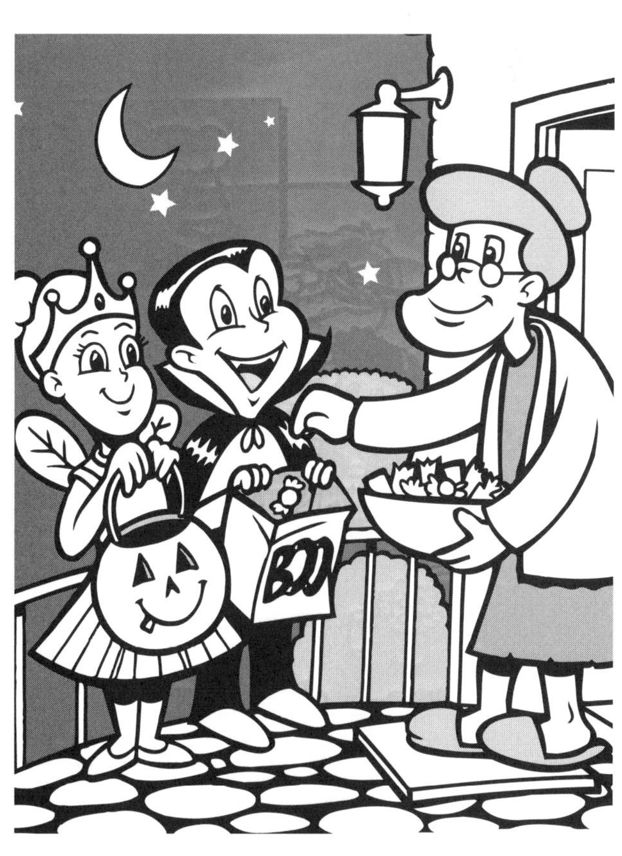

1 2 3 4

- ***Who*** is not in a costume?
- ***What*** are the costumes?

- ***Where*** do children trick or treat?
- ***When*** do you wear a costume?

- ***Why*** does the lady have a bowl full of candy?
- ***How*** do we thank people when they give us something?

Hanukkah

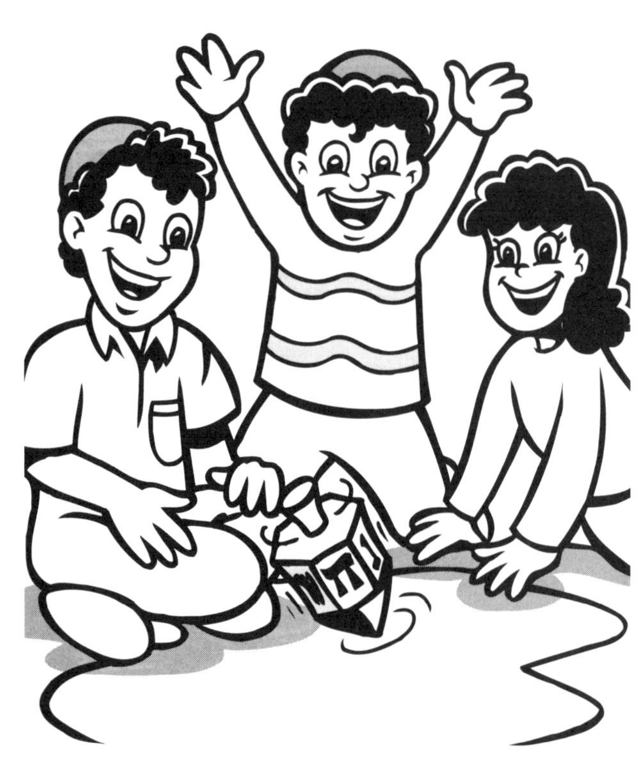

- ***Who*** is spinning the dreidel?
- ***What*** are these children spinning?

- ***Where*** is the dreidel?
- ***When*** do children play games?

- ***Why*** do children take turns?
- ***How*** do you play with a dreidel?

Cut on dotted line

Cut on dotted line

- ***When*** do people celebrate Kwanzaa?
- ***What*** are they lighting?
- ***Where*** is the Kinara (candle holder)?
- ***Who*** is helping the boy?

1 2 3 4

Kwanzaa

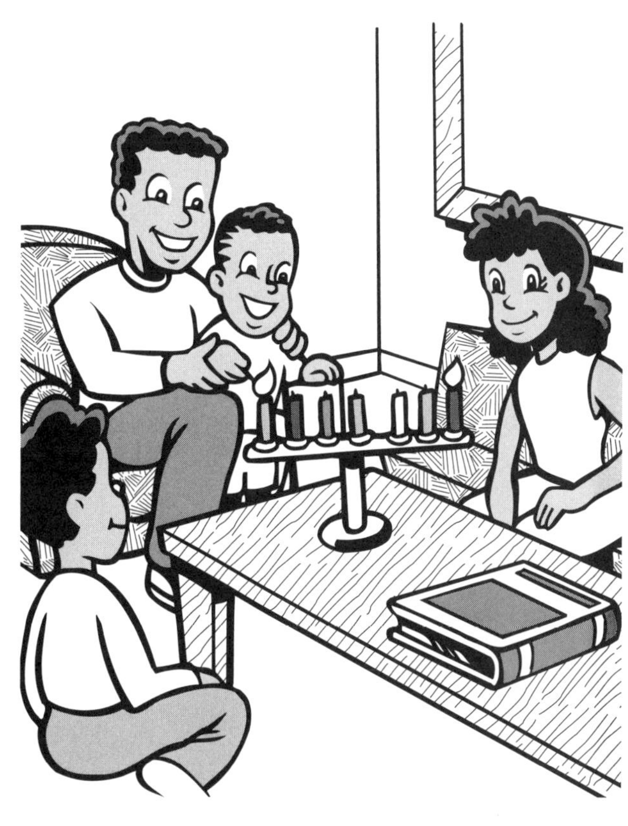

- ***Why*** is the father helping the boy?
- ***How*** do you light a candle?

- ***When*** did he give this speech?
- ***Where*** is he standing?

- ***What*** is he saying?
- ***Who*** is giving the speech?

2 3
4 1

Martin Luther King, Jr.

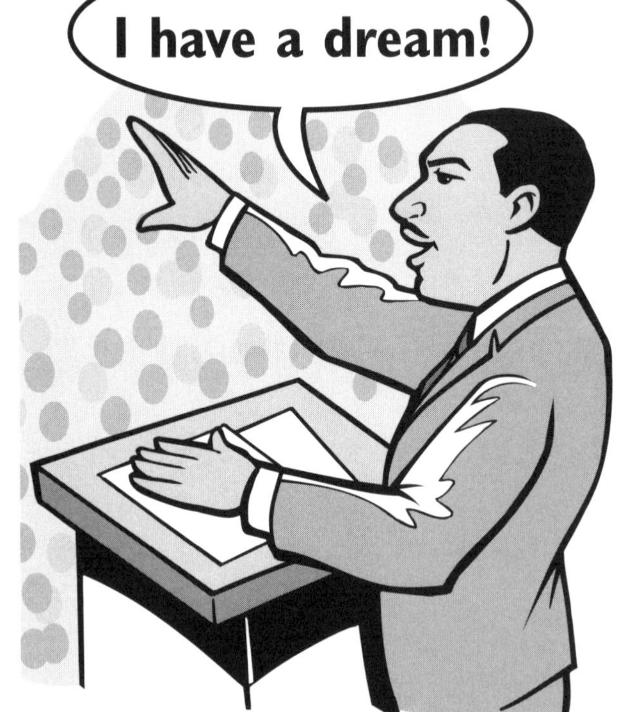
I have a dream!

- ***Why*** are there so many people watching him?
- ***How*** do you write a speech?

Cut on dotted line

Cut on dotted line

Mother's Day

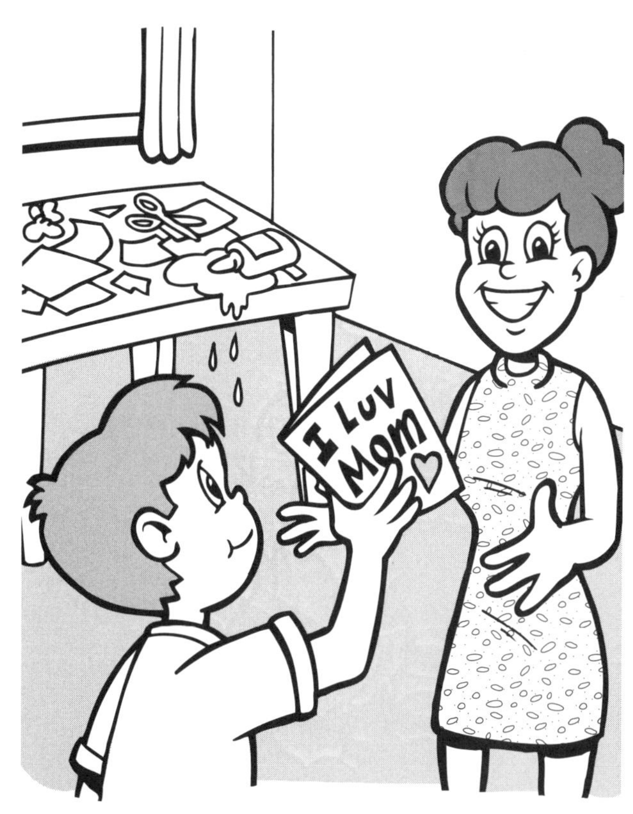

1 2 3 4

- ***Who*** is receiving the card?
- ***What*** is the child giving his mother?
- ***Where*** did the boy make this card?
- ***When*** do you give your mother a card?
- ***Why*** is this mother smiling?
- ***How*** did the child make this card?

Cut on dotted line

New Baby

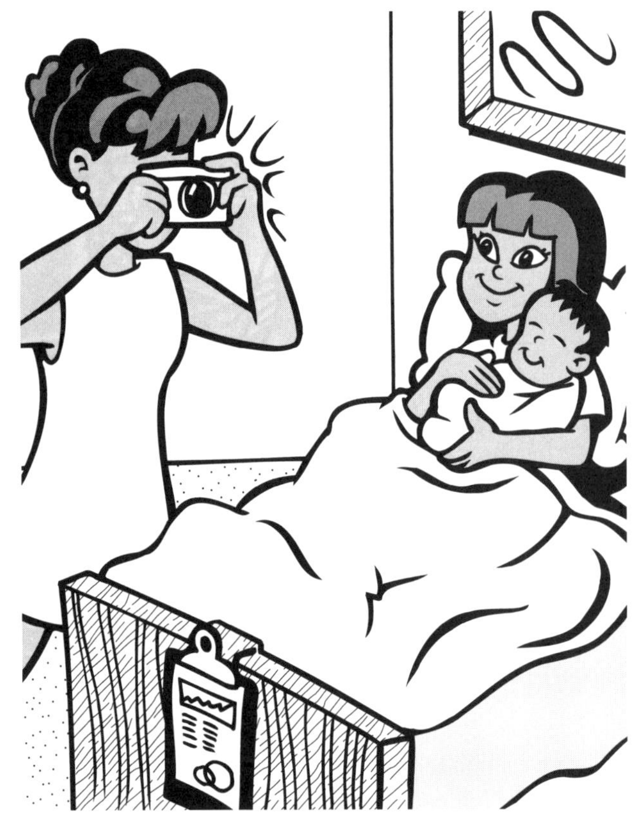

- ***Who*** is in bed?
- ***What*** is this mother holding?

- ***Where*** are these people?
- ***When*** do babies cry?

- ***Why*** do people take pictures of new babies?

- ***How*** do people keep babies warm?

1 2 3 4

New Year's

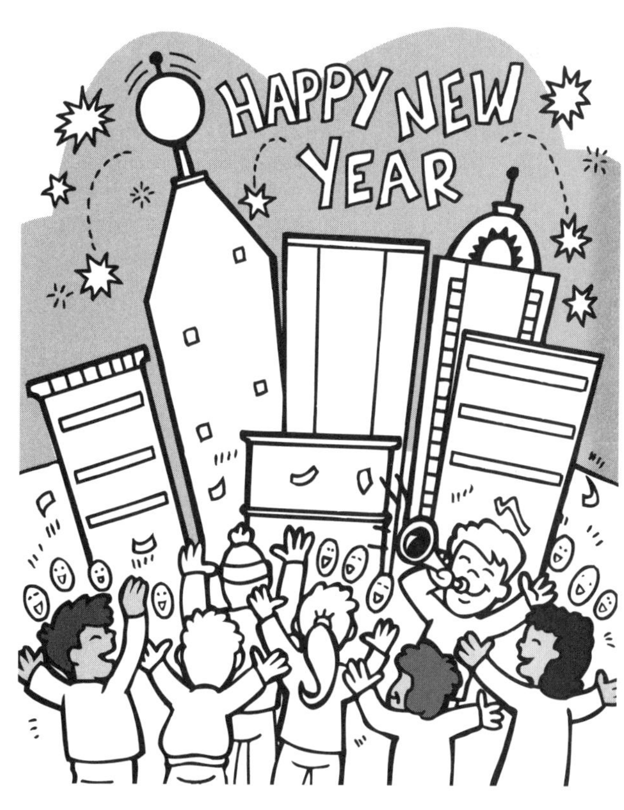

1 2 3 4

- ***Who*** celebrates New Year's Day?
- ***What*** is going down the pole on the building?
- ***Where*** is this crowd?
- ***When*** do you have celebrations?
- ***Why*** are these people excited?
- ***How*** do you have fun on New Year's Day?

Planting/Watering

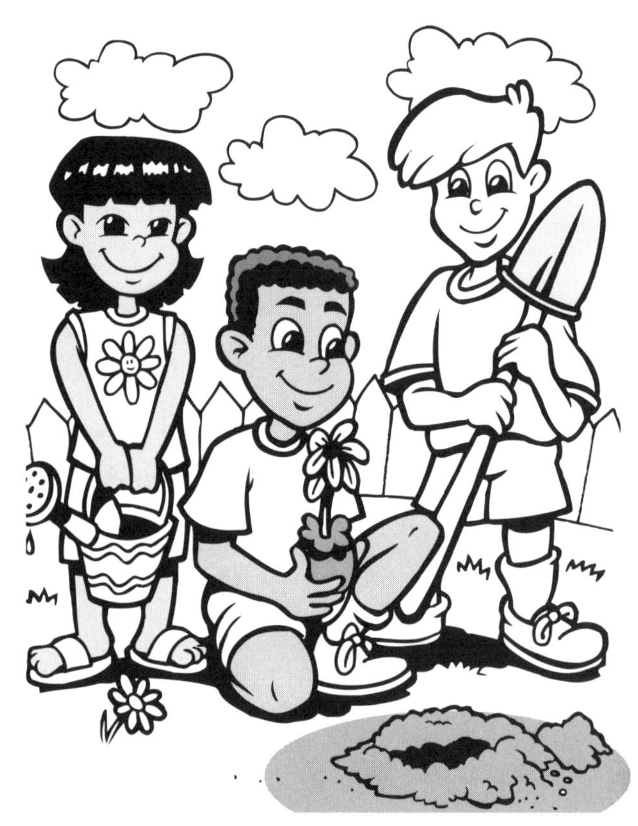

- ***Who*** has the watering can?

- ***What*** are these children planting?

- ***Where*** are flowers planted?

- ***When*** do flowers bloom?

- ***Why*** do flowers need water?

- ***How*** do people water flowers?

Cut on dotted line

Cut on dotted line

1 2 3 4

President's Day

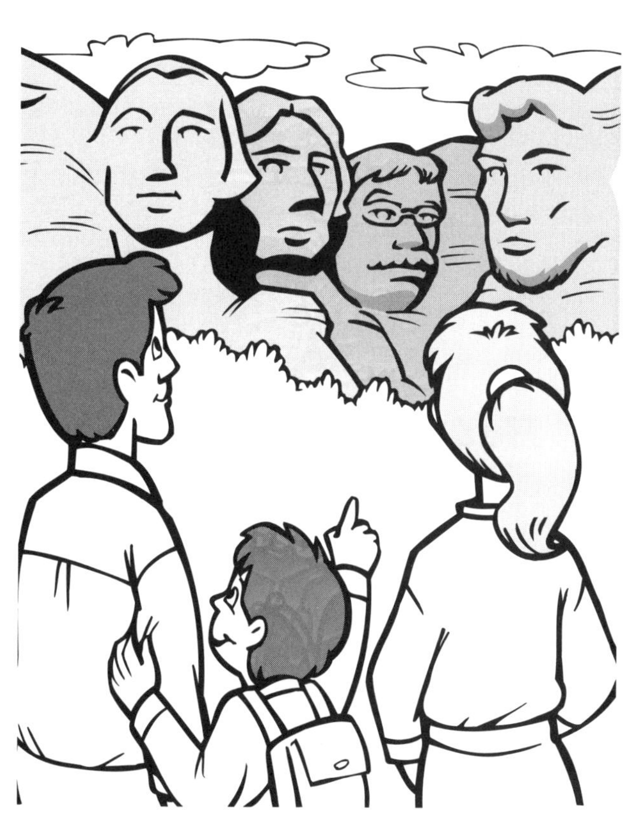

- ***Who*** is in the sculpture?
- ***What*** is the sculpture made of?

- ***Where*** is the family?
- ***When*** will they go home?

- ***Why*** is the boy pointing?
- ***How*** did this sculpture get on this mountain?

Raking Leaves

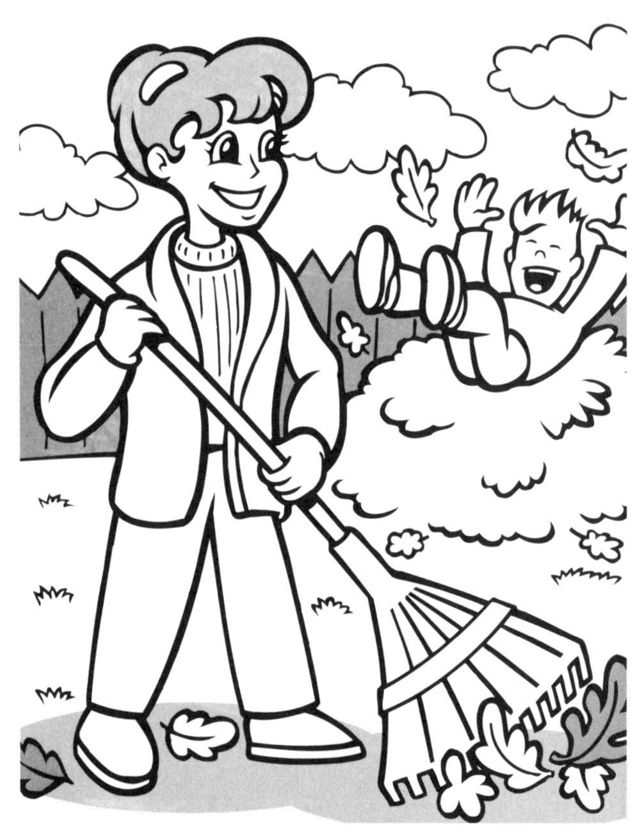

- ***Who*** is in the leaf pile?
- ***What*** does the lady have in her hand?
- ***Where*** do leaves fall?
- ***When*** do leaves fall?
- ***Why*** do people rake leaves?
- ***How*** do you make a pile of leaves?

Cut on dotted line

Saint Patrick's Day

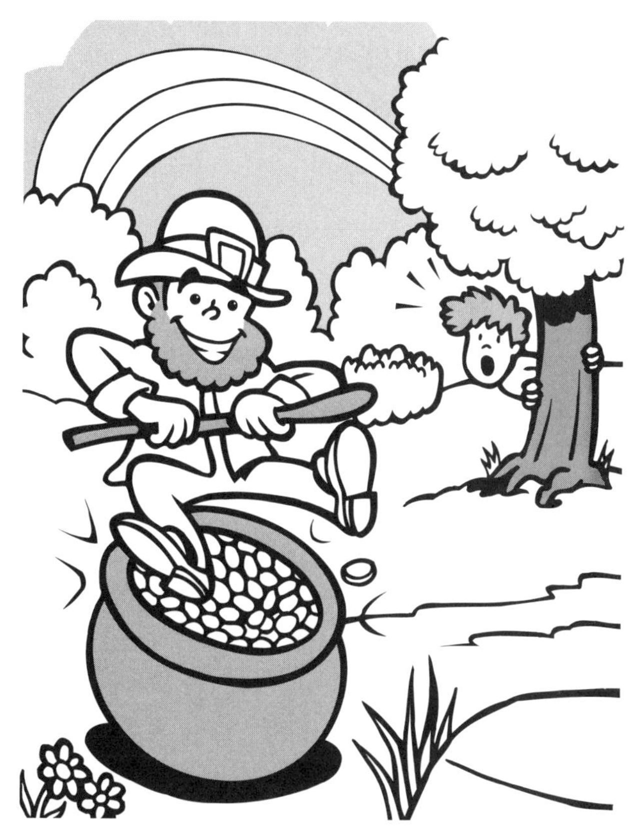

- ***Who*** is watching the leprechaun?
- ***What*** does the leprechaun have?

- ***Where*** is the child hiding?
- ***When*** is Saint Patrick's Day?

- ***Why*** is the child hiding?
- ***How*** much gold is in the pot?

Cut on dotted line

1 2 3 4

Sledding

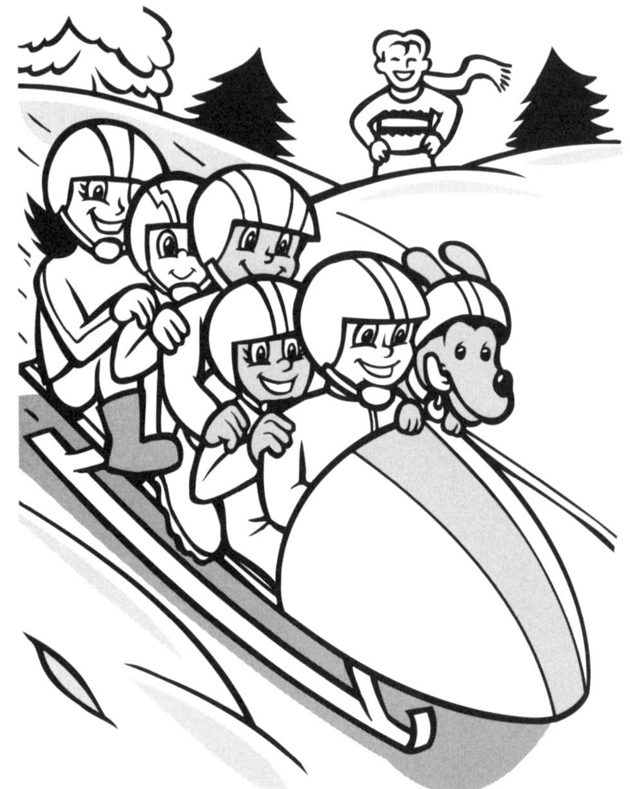

- ***Who*** is watching the children?
- ***What*** are these children sitting on?

- ***Where*** are these children going?
- ***When*** would a child go sledding?

- ***Why*** are these children wearing helmets?

- ***How*** many children fit on this sled?

Cut on dotted line

Snowman

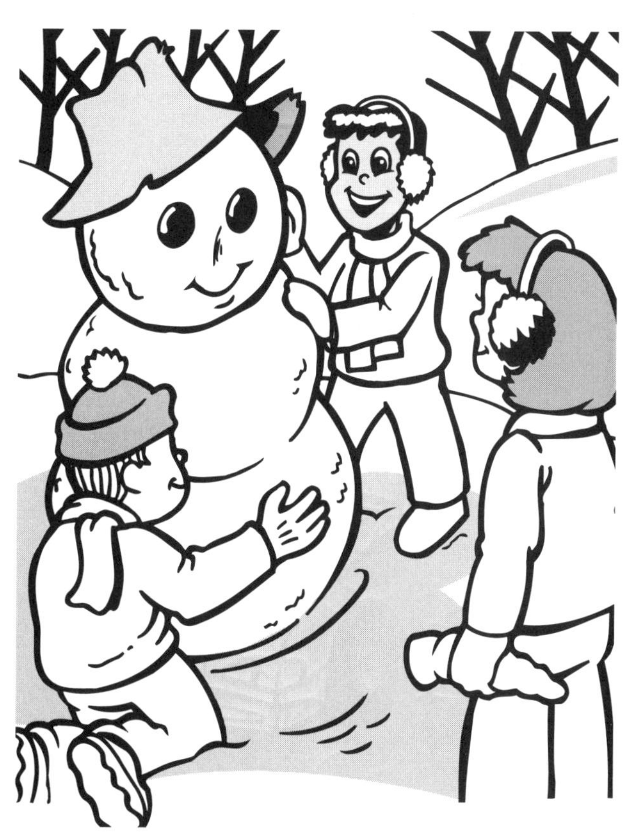

- ***Who*** has the carrot?
- ***What*** are the children making?

- ***Where*** do people make snowmen?
- ***When*** will the snowman melt?

- ***Why*** do children wear warm clothes in winter?
- ***How*** do you make a snowman?

Cut on dotted line

Summer at the Pool

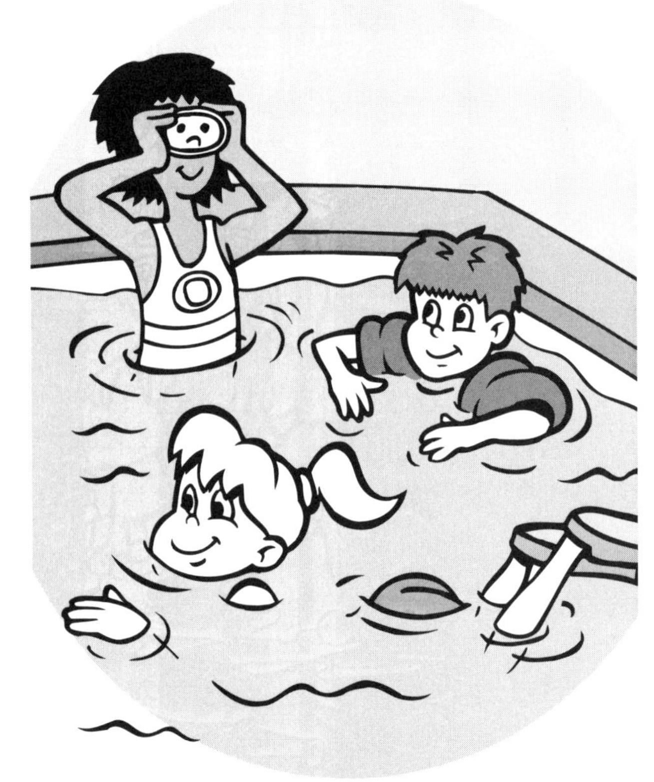

- ***Who*** is wearing goggles?
- ***What*** is the smallest child wearing?

- ***Where*** are these children?
- ***When*** do children need to wear floaties?

- ***Why*** do people wear flippers?
- ***How*** do goggles stay on someone's eyes?

1 2 3 4

Thanksgiving

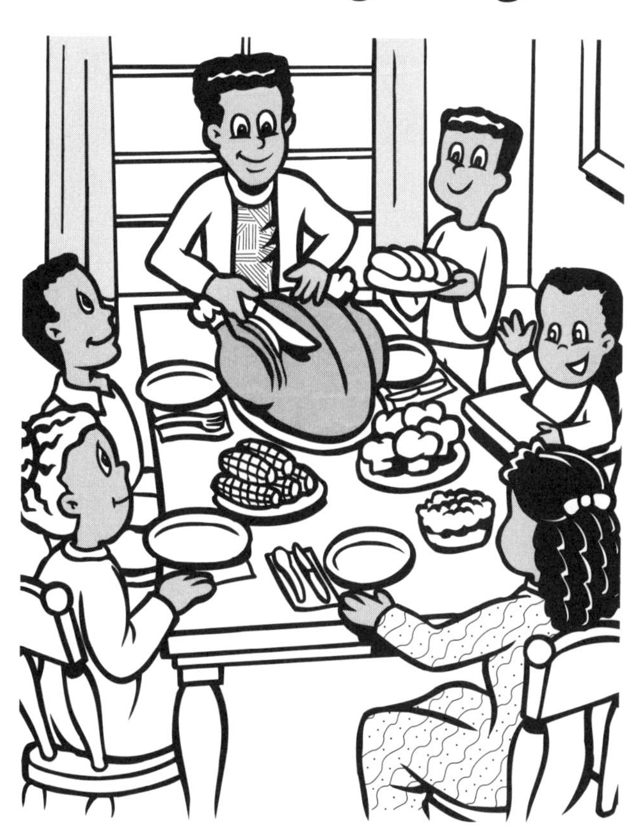

- ***Who*** is carving the turkey?
- ***What*** is on the table?

- ***Where*** is the baby sitting?
- ***When*** will these people eat?

- ***Why*** is Thanksgiving celebrated with a meal?
- ***How*** much food do you eat on Thanksgiving Day?

Cut on dotted line

Cut on dotted line

1

Tooth Fairy

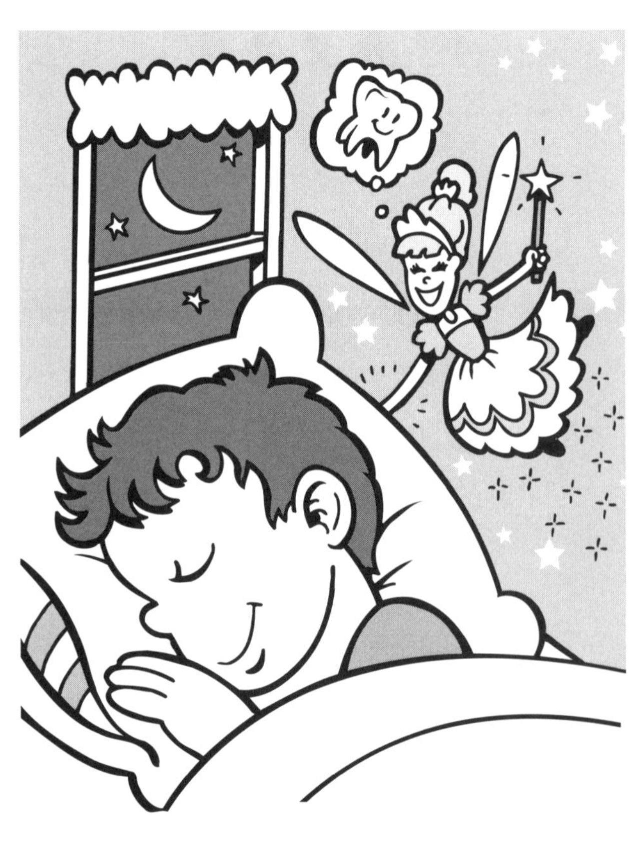

2

- ***Who*** is in the room with the boy?
- ***What*** is the tooth fairy reaching for?

3

- ***Where*** will she put the surprise?
- ***When*** does the tooth fairy visit you?

4

- ***Why*** doesn't the tooth fairy visit every night?
- ***How*** does the tooth fairy find the tooth without waking up the child?

Cut on dotted line

- ***When*** do people receive valentines?

- ***What*** is in the boy's hand?

- ***Where*** are the flowers?

- ***Who*** is giving a valentine?

2 3
1 4

- ***Why*** does the boy have flowers?

- ***How*** does this girl feel?

Valentine's Day

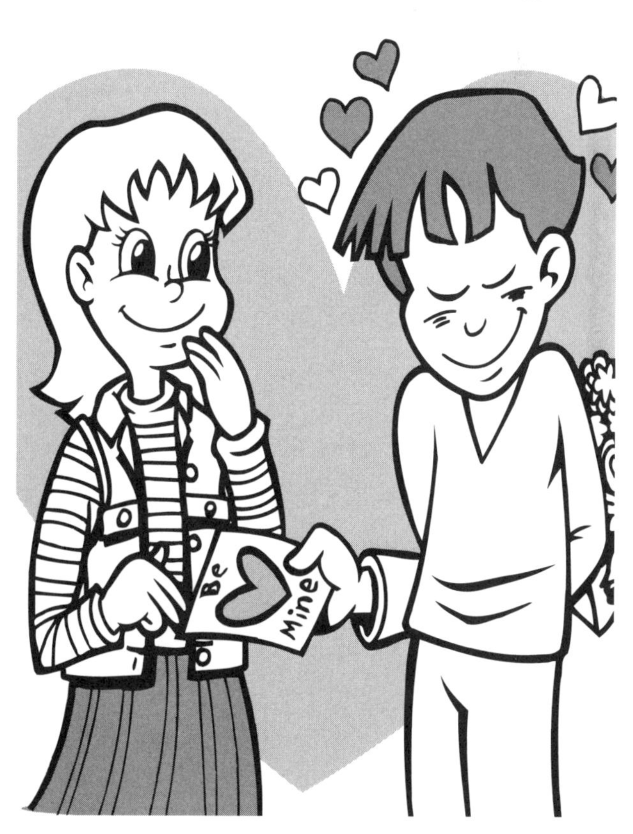

Cut on dotted line

1 2 3 4

Wedding

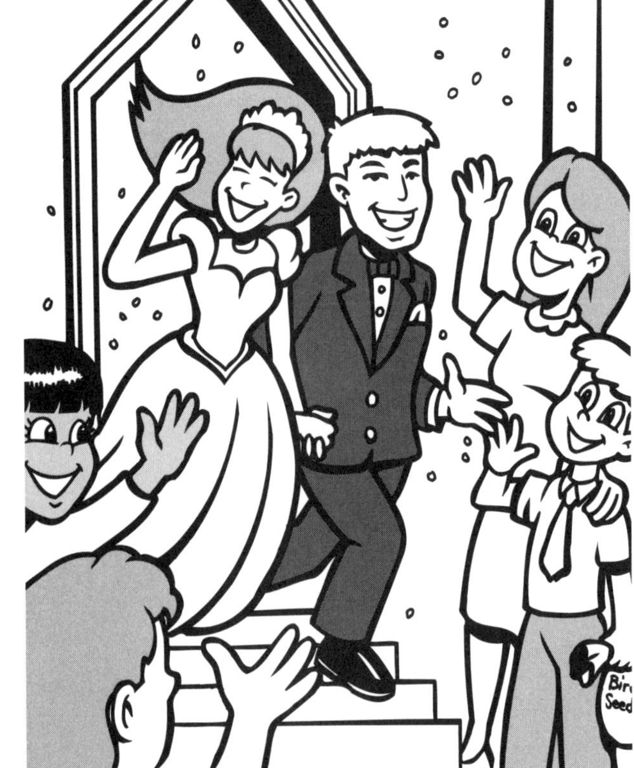

- ***Who*** is wearing a dress?
- ***What*** are the people throwing on the newlyweds?

- ***Where*** are the newlyweds going?
- ***When*** do the bride and groom kiss at a wedding?

- ***Why*** do people go to weddings?
- ***How*** will the newlyweds get home?

Home

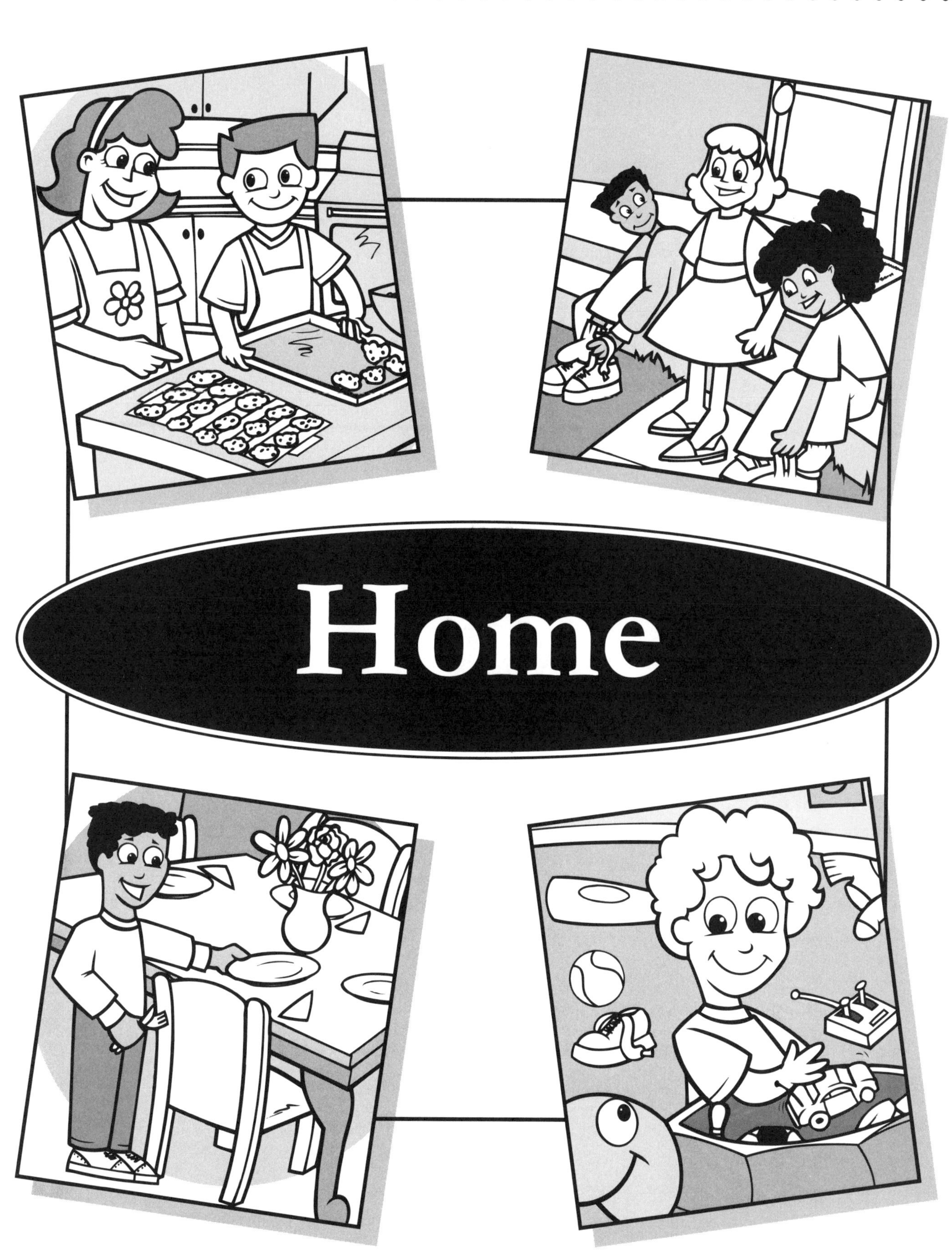

Cut on dotted line

Home

Baking Cookies

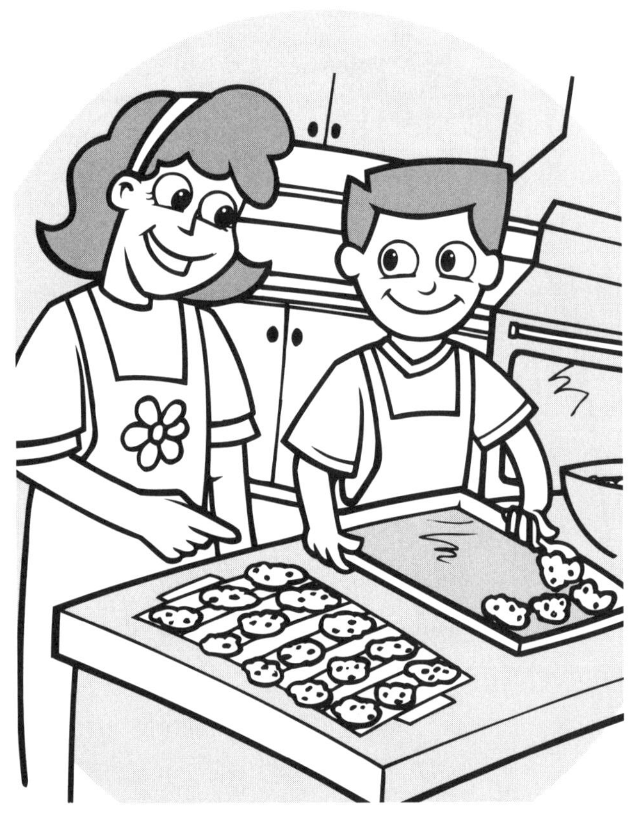

- ***Who*** is making cookies?

- ***What*** kind of cookies are they making?

- ***Where*** do you bake cookies?

- ***When*** do you take the cookies out of the oven?

- ***Why*** is the mother helping the boy?

- ***How*** do you know when the cookies are done?

Cut on dotted line

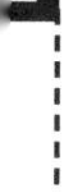

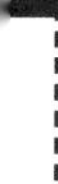
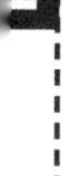

Home

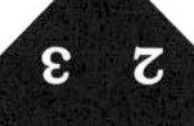
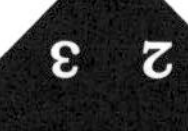

1 2 3 4

Bath Time

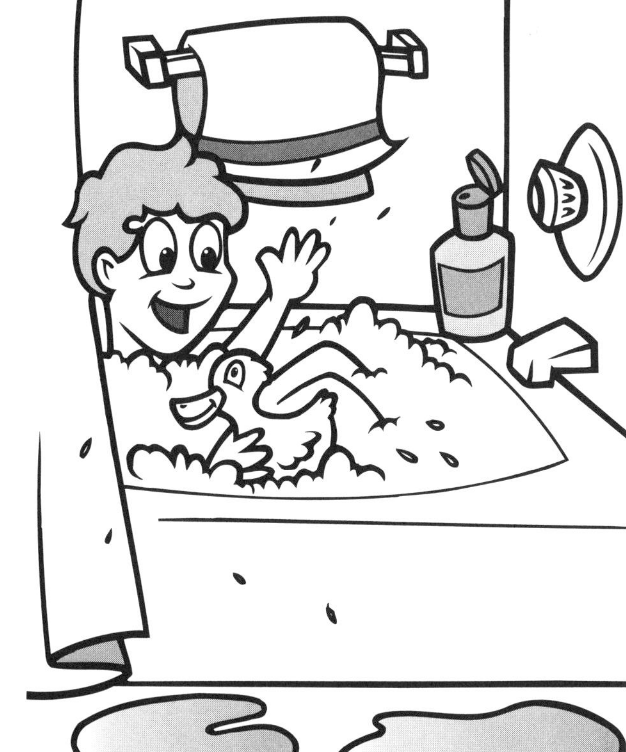

- ***Who*** is in the tub?
- ***What*** is in the tub with him?

- ***Where*** is the water?
- ***When*** do you take a bath?

- ***Why*** is he splashing?
- ***How*** will he dry off?

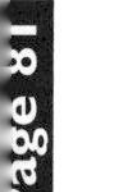

1 2
4 3

Bedtime

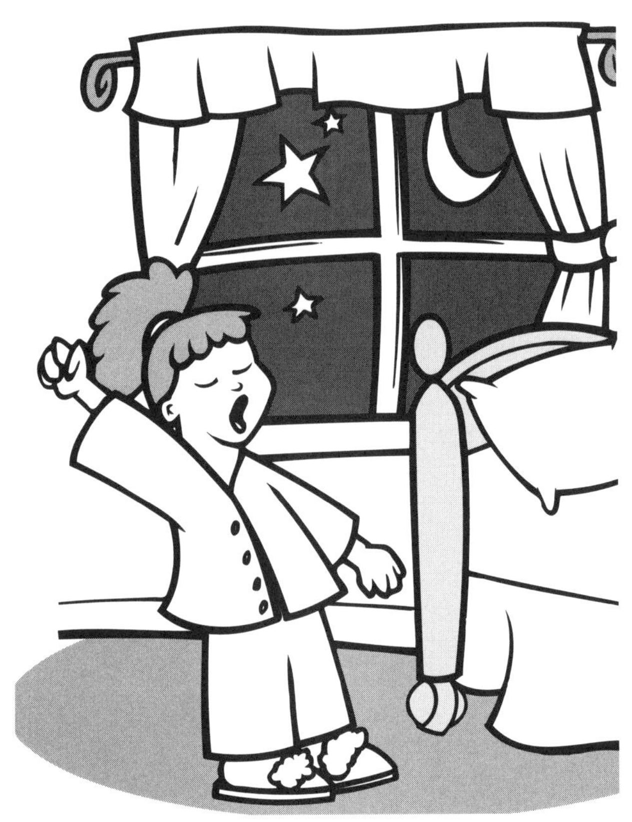

- ***Who*** is going to bed?
- ***What*** does she wear at bedtime?

- ***Where*** does she sleep?
- ***When*** do you go to bed?

- ***Why*** do you sleep?
- ***How*** do you get ready for bed?

Cut on dotted line

Brushing Teeth

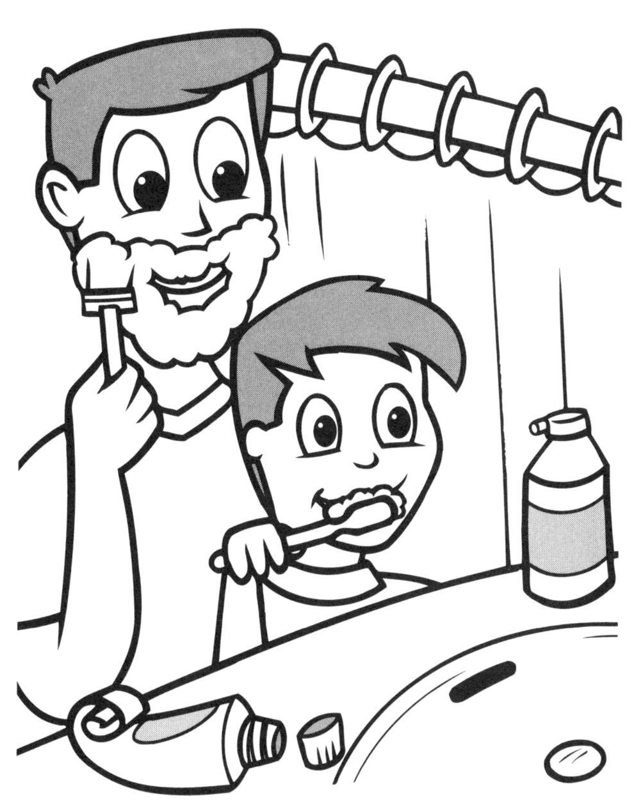

1 2 3 4

- **Who** is shaving?

- **What** does the boy have in his hand?

- **Where** are they?

- **When** do you brush your teeth?

- ***Why*** does a toothbrush have a long handle?

- ***How*** do you rinse your teeth?

Cleaning the Room

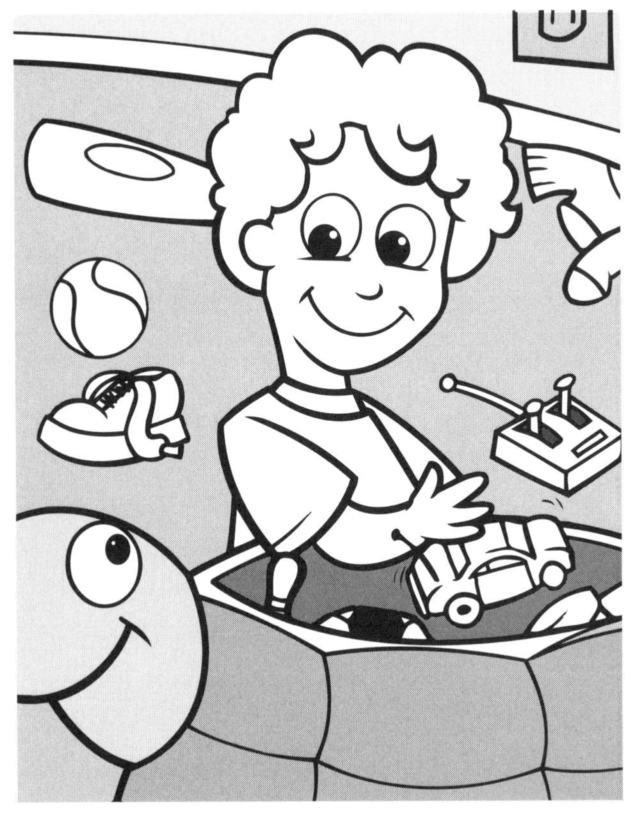

- ***Who*** is cleaning the room?
- ***What*** is the child carrying?

- ***Where*** is the toy chest?
- ***When*** do you clean your room?

- ***Why*** do you put toys away?
- ***How*** do you clean your room?

Cut on dotted line

Home

Dinnertime

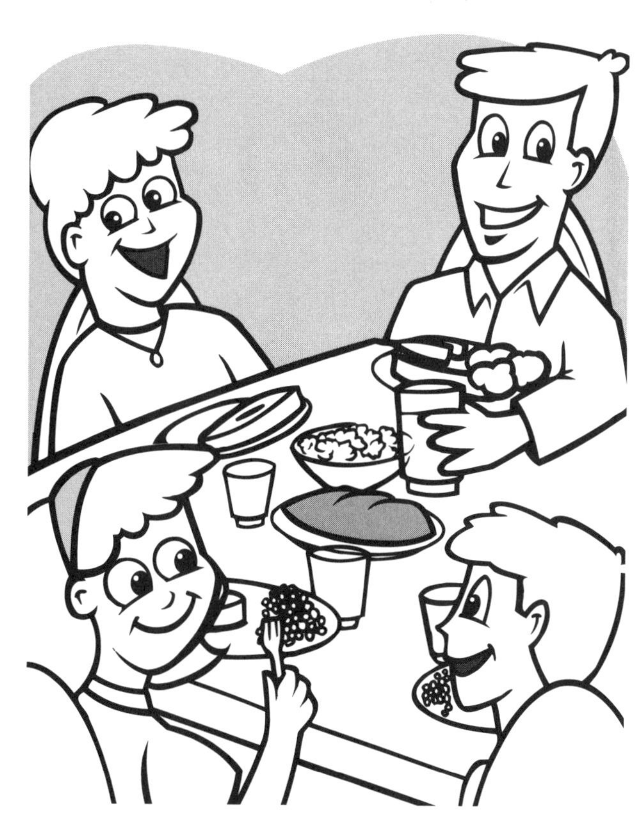

- ***Who*** is eating the dinner?
- ***What*** are they eating?
- ***Where*** are they sitting?
- ***When*** do you eat dinner?
- ***Why*** are these people smiling?
- ***How*** do you ask for more food?

1 2 3 4

Dressing

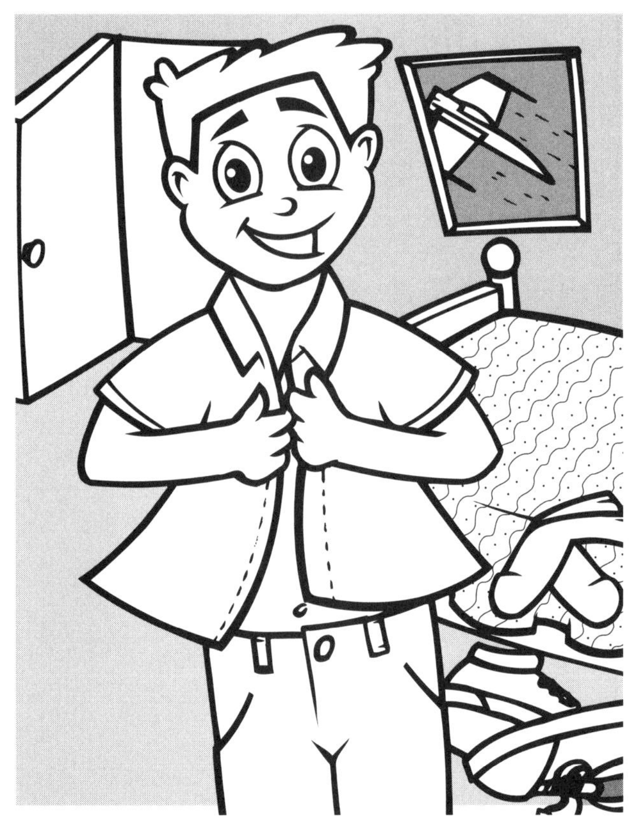

- ***Who*** is getting ready?
- ***What*** is he putting on?

- ***Where*** are his shoes and socks?
- ***When*** do you get dressed?

- ***Why*** do we wear clothes?
- ***How*** do you get dressed?

1 2 3 4

Cut on dotted line

Feeding the Dog

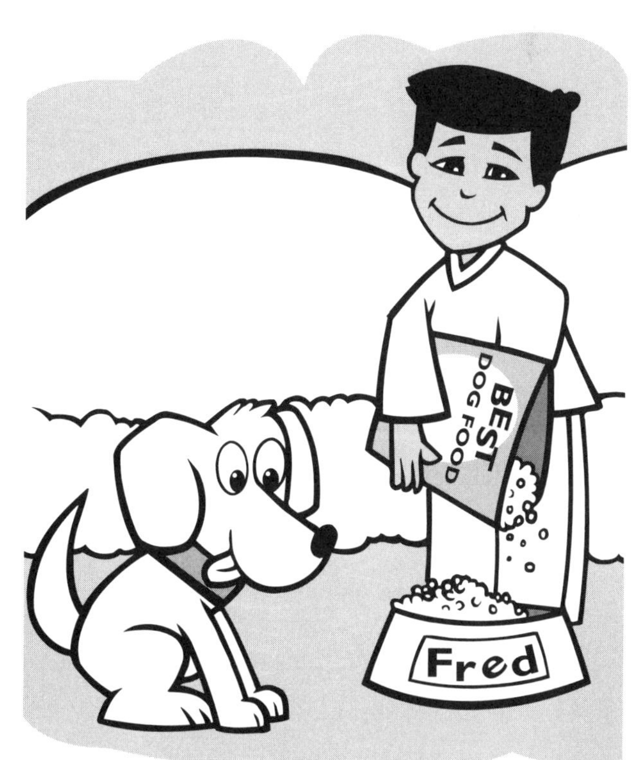

- ***Who*** is feeding the dog?

- ***What*** does the dog eat?

- ***Where*** does the dog eat?

- ***When*** do you feed a dog?

- ***Why*** does the dog have his own food?

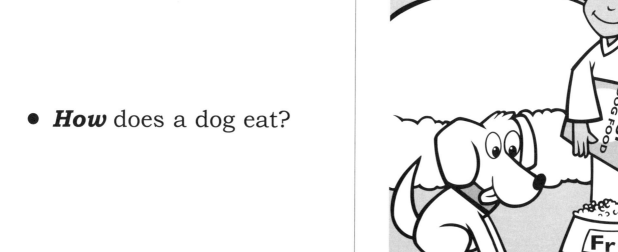

- ***How*** does a dog eat?

Cut on dotted line

Retrieving the Mail

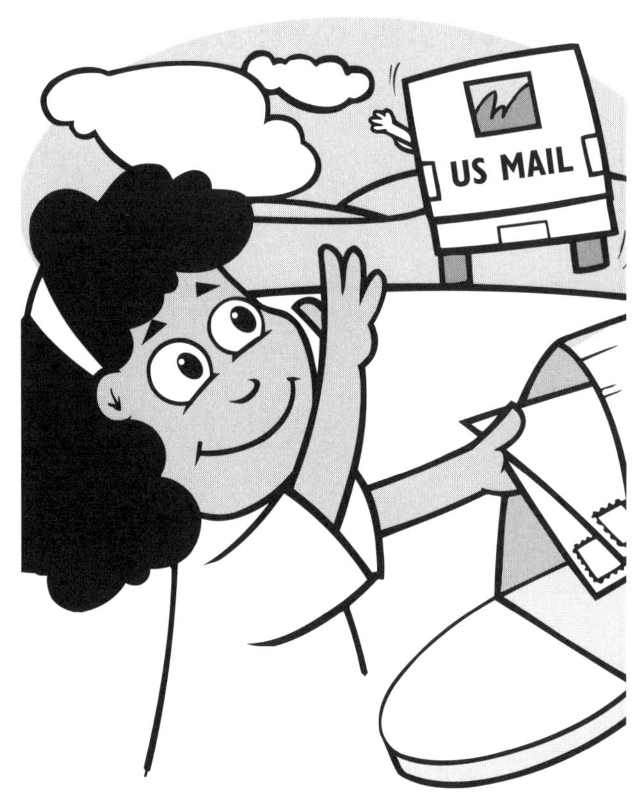

- ***Who*** is the girl waving to?
- ***What*** is she holding?

- ***Where*** does the mail carrier put the mail?
- ***When*** do people get letters?

- ***Why*** is the girl happy?
- ***How*** do you send a letter?

Sending Mail

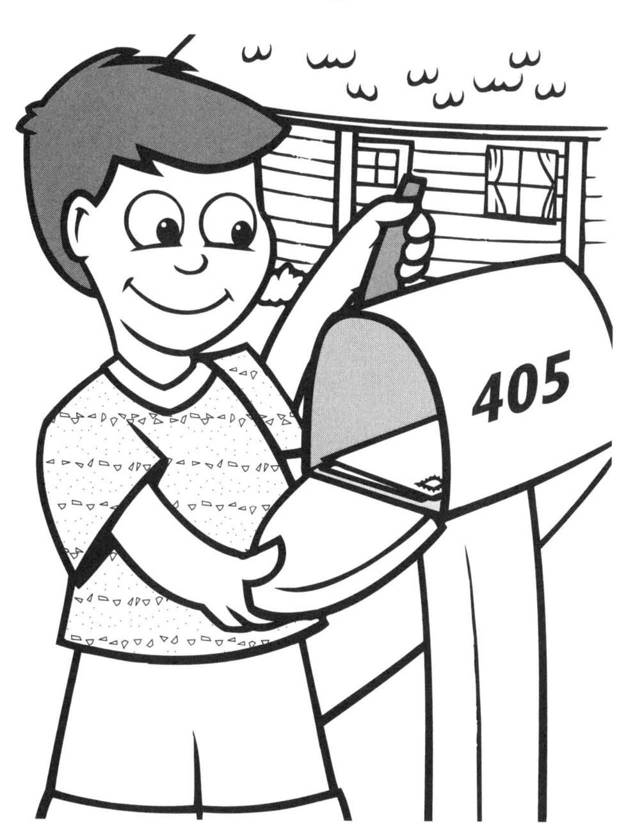

- ***Who*** is mailing the letter?
- ***What*** is he putting it in?
- ***Where*** will the mail carrier take the letter?
- ***When*** will the boy know the letter has been picked up?
- ***Why*** is he putting the flag up?
- ***How*** does the post office know where to send the letter?

Cut on dotted line

Home

Cut on dotted line

Setting the Table

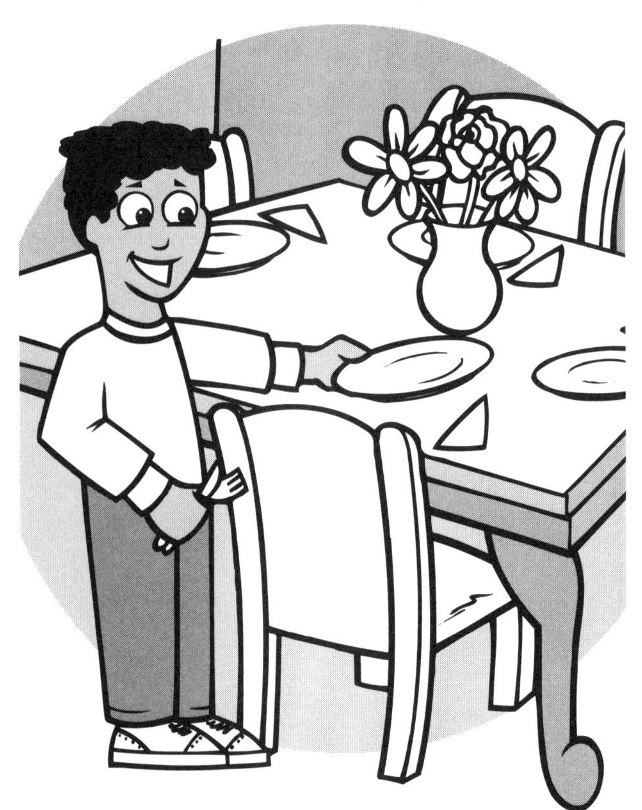

- ***Who*** is setting the table?
- ***What*** does he have in his hand?

- ***Where*** are the flowers?
- ***When*** do you set the table?

- ***Why*** are there four places at the table?
- ***How*** do you get ready for a meal?

Cut on dotted line

Home

Sweeping the Porch

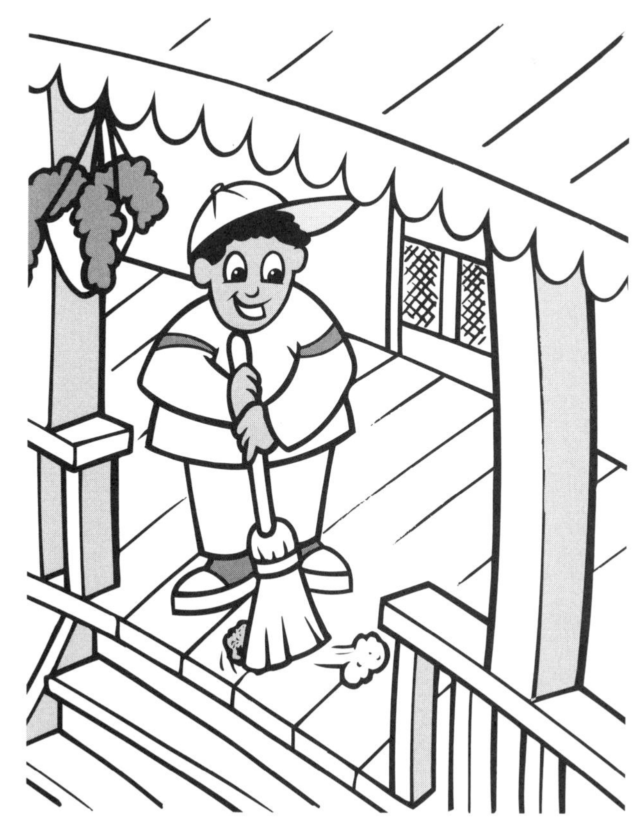

1 2 3 4

- ***Who*** is sweeping the porch?
- ***What*** do you sweep with?

- ***Where*** do you find a porch?
- ***When*** do you sweep?

- ***Why*** do you need to sweep?
- ***How*** do you sweep a porch?

Cut on dotted line

Taking Out the Trash

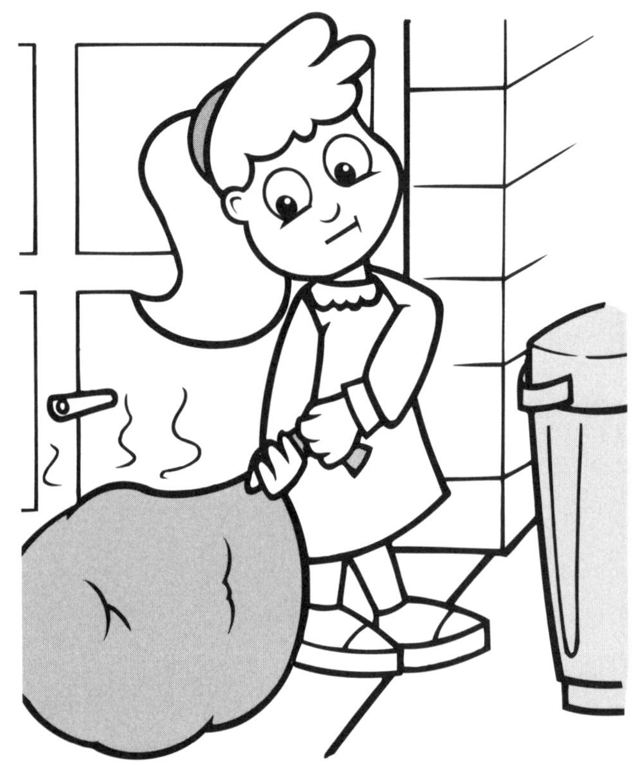

- ***Who*** is taking out the trash?
- ***What*** is in the trash bag?

- ***Where*** does the trash go?
- ***When*** do you take out the trash?

- ***Why*** does the girl have that look on her face?
- ***How*** does the trash get to the dump?

1 2 3 4

Tying Shoes

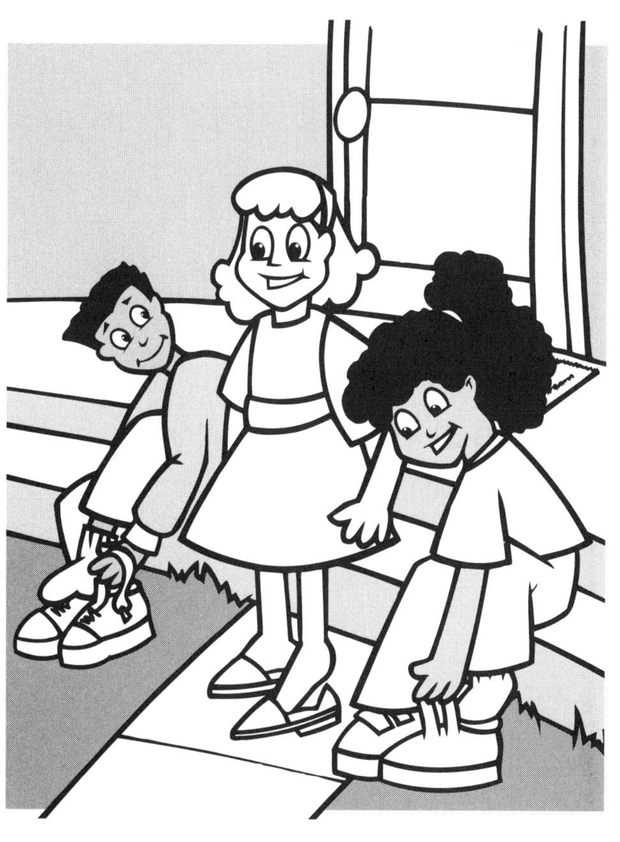

- ***Who*** has shoestrings to tie?
- ***What*** do the children have on their feet?
- ***Where*** do you wear shoes?
- ***When*** do you take your shoes off?
- ***Why*** do people wear shoes?
- ***How*** many different shoes do you have?

1 2 3 4

Waking Up

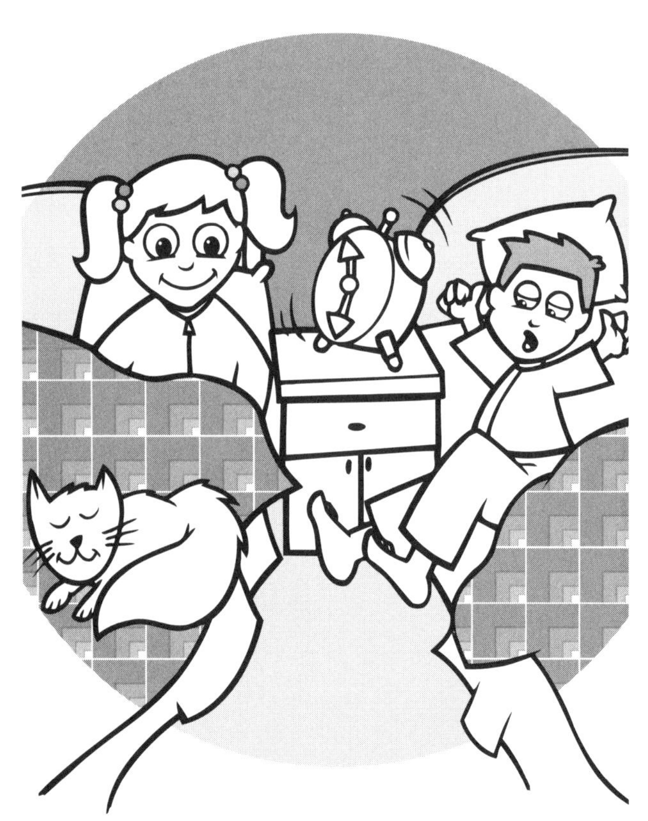

- ***Who*** is sleeping?
- ***What*** is on the bed?

- ***Where*** are the children sleeping?
- ***When*** do you wake up?

- ***Why*** do you sleep?
- ***How*** early do you wake up?

1 2 3 4

Cut on dotted line

Home

Cut on dotted line

Washing Dishes

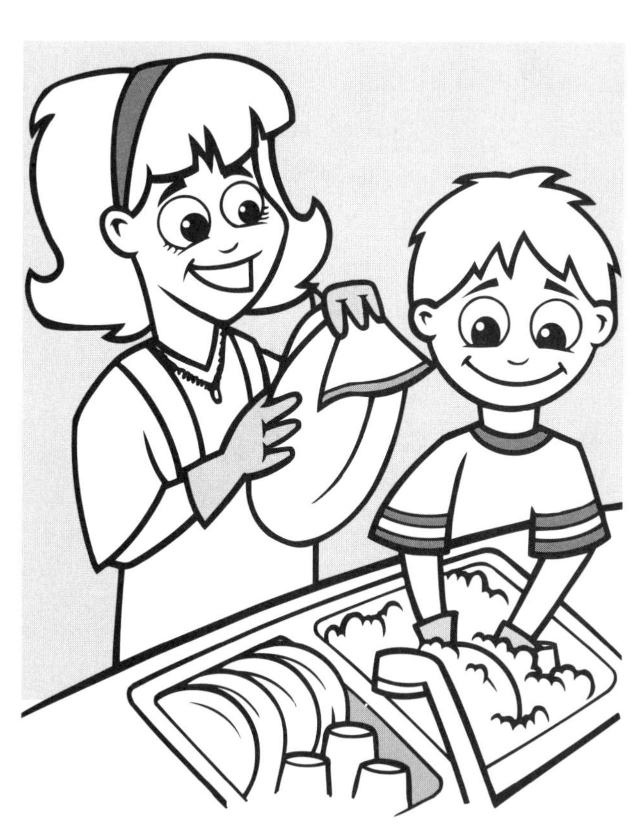

- ***Who*** is washing the dishes?
- ***What*** is the mother holding?

- ***Where*** do you wash dishes?
- ***When*** do you do the dishes?

- ***Why*** do dishes need to be clean?
- ***How*** do dishes get dirty?

1 2 3 4

Cut on dotted line

Home

Watching TV

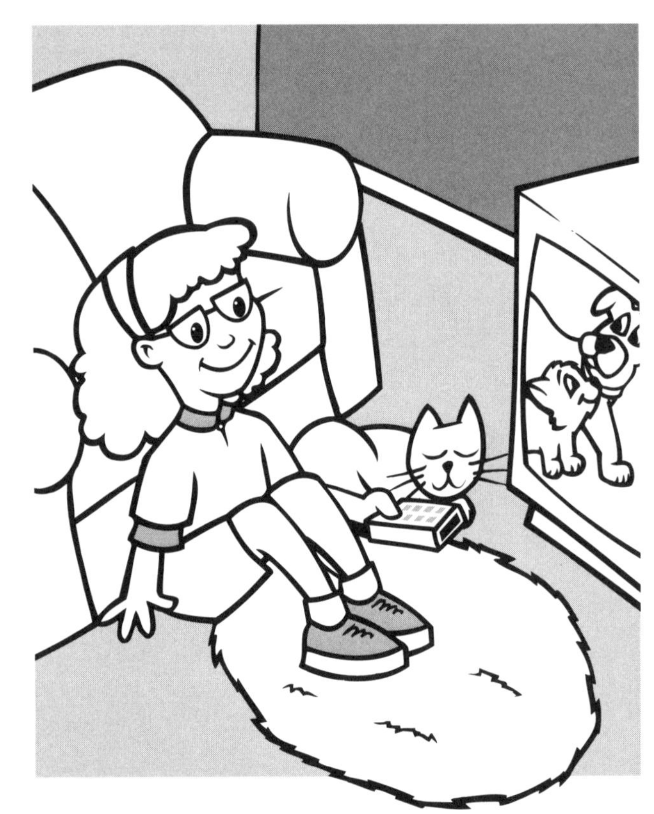

- ***Who*** is watching TV?
- ***What*** type of show is she watching?
- ***Where*** is she sitting?
- ***When*** do you watch TV?
- ***Why*** is she smiling?
- ***How*** will the girl change TV channels?

Working on Homework

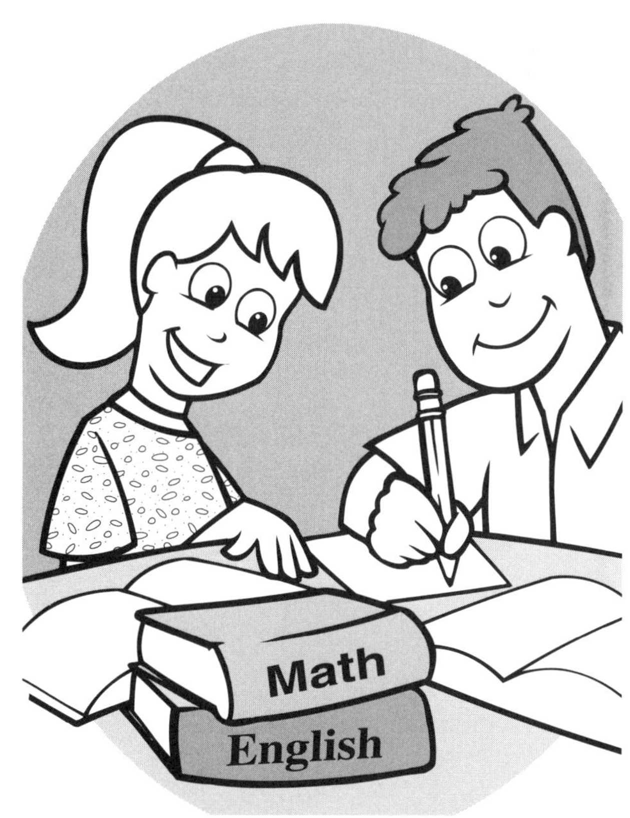

- ***Who*** is holding the pencil?

- ***What*** is he writing on?

- ***Where*** are they working?

- ***When*** do you do homework?

- ***Why*** do you do school work at home?

- ***How*** do you know what to work on at home?

Cut on dotted line

Writing a Letter

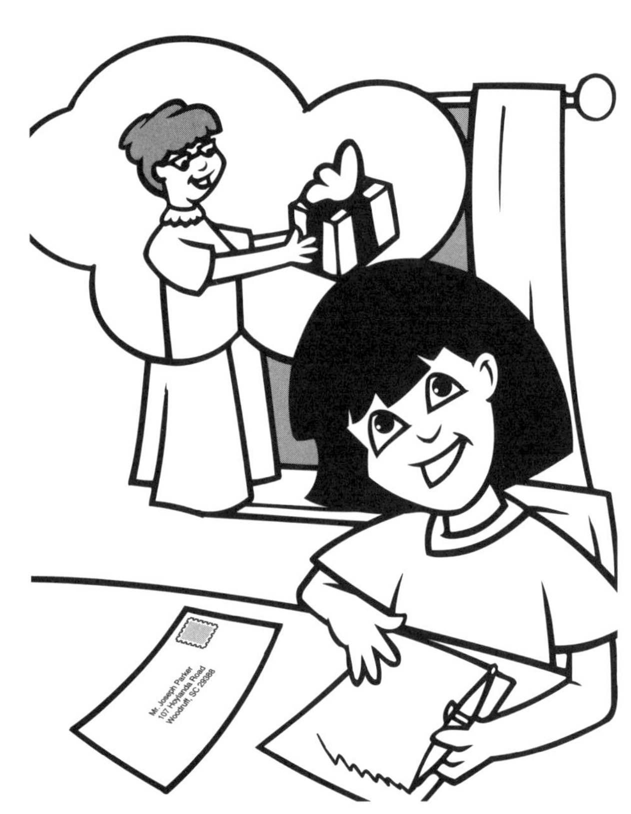

- ***Who*** is she writing a letter to?
- ***What*** is she writing with?
- ***Where*** is the envelope?
- ***When*** will she mail the letter?
- ***Why*** is she writing a letter?
- ***How*** do you write a letter?

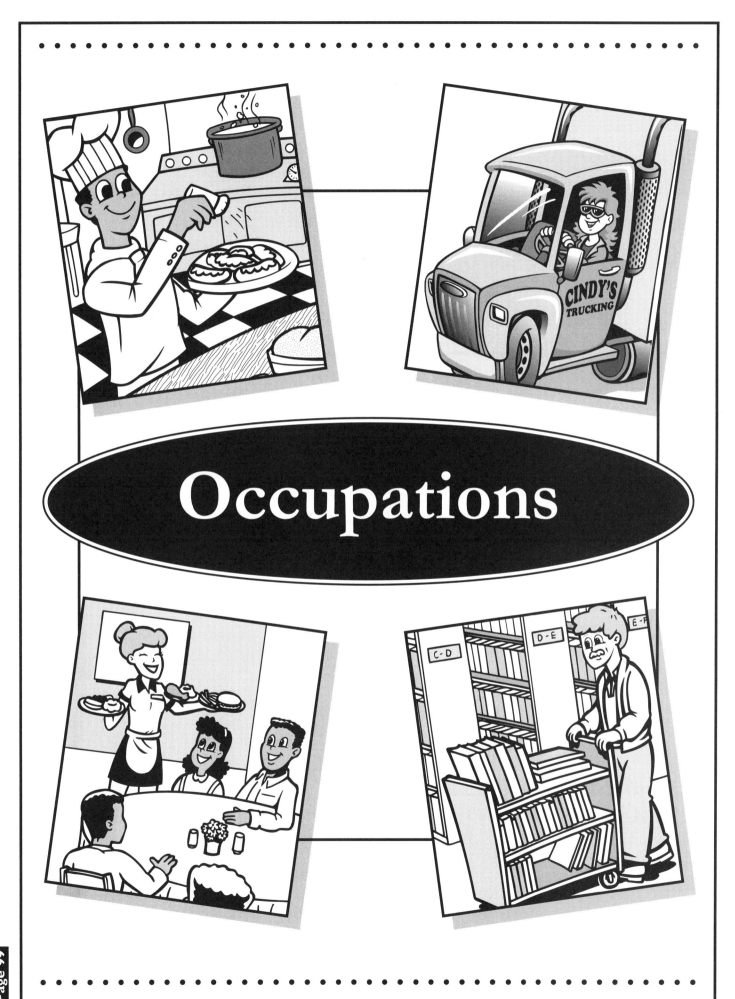
Occupations
CINDY'S
TRUCKING
C-D
D-E

Cut on dotted line

Occupations

Audiologist

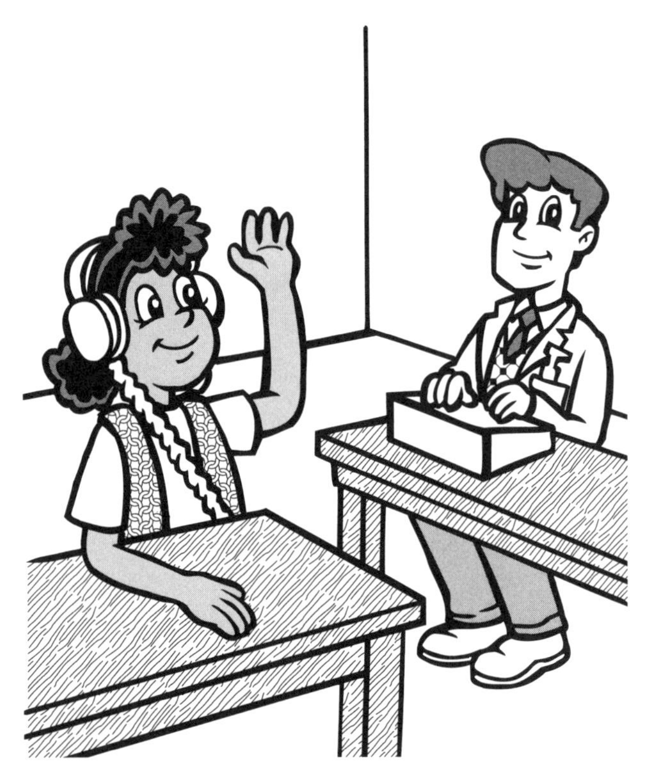

- ***Who*** tests people's hearing?
- ***What*** do people wear for a hearing test?

- ***Where*** does this person work?
- ***When*** should hearing be tested?

- ***Why*** is hearing important?

- ***How*** does this person look into your ears?

Cut on dotted line

- ***What*** is the bank teller holding?
- ***Who*** is in the car?
- ***When*** do people go to the bank?
- ***Where*** are these people?

2 3
1 4

Bank Teller

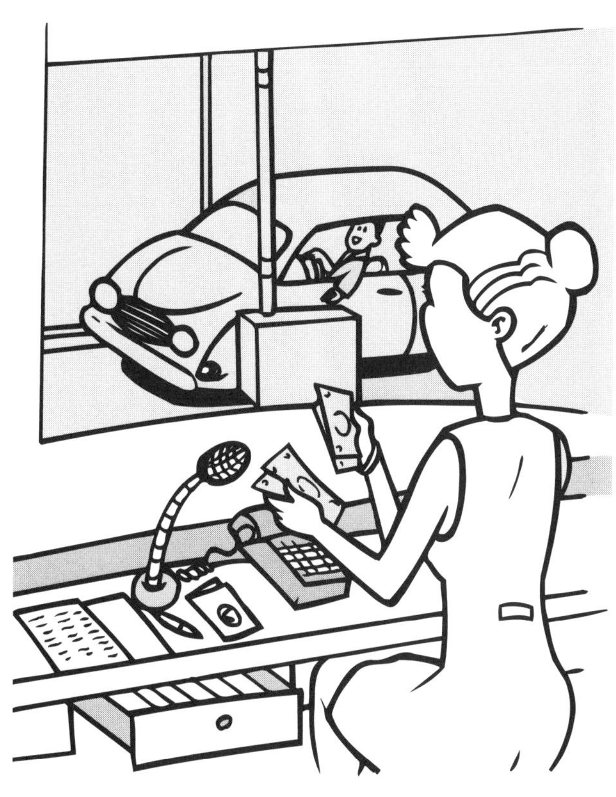

- ***Why*** is counting important to a bank teller?
- ***How*** does the bank teller at the window get money to the person in the car?

Bellboy

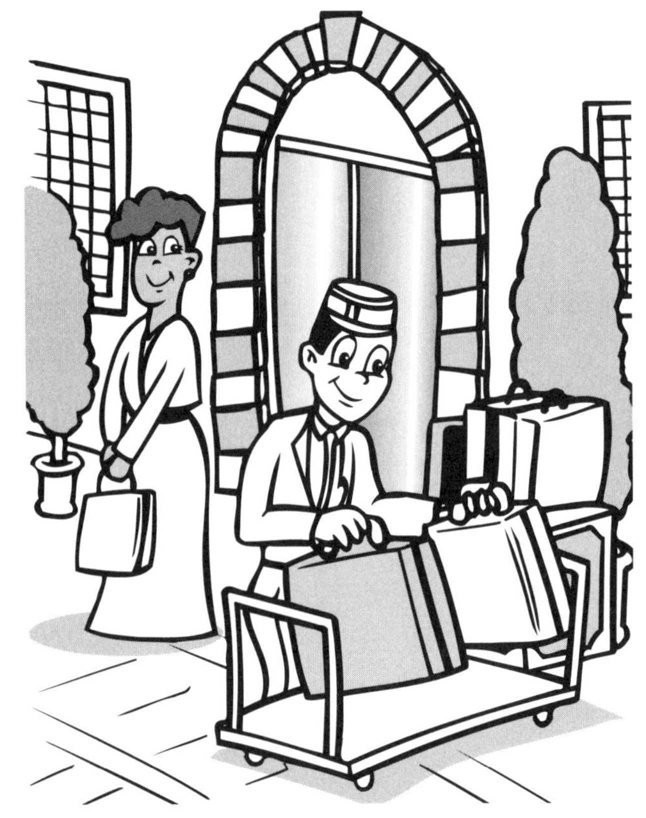

- ***Who*** is helping this lady?
- ***What*** is the bellboy putting on the cart?

- ***Where*** will he take her luggage?
- ***When*** do people tip bellboys?

- ***Why*** do bellboys use carts?
- ***How*** does a bellboy treat a visitor?

Cut on dotted line

Cut on dotted line

- ***When*** do people go to restaurants?

- ***What*** does he have on his head?

- ***Where*** do you cook?

- ***Who*** cooks the food in a fancy restaurant?

Occupations

2 3
1 4

Chef

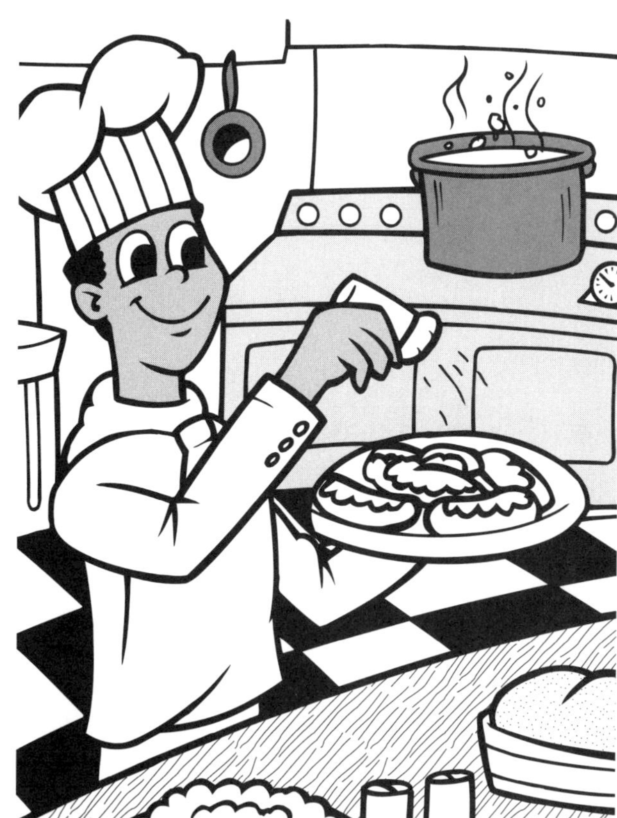

- ***Why*** does the chef add seasonings to food?

- ***How*** do you know when food is ready to eat?

Doctor

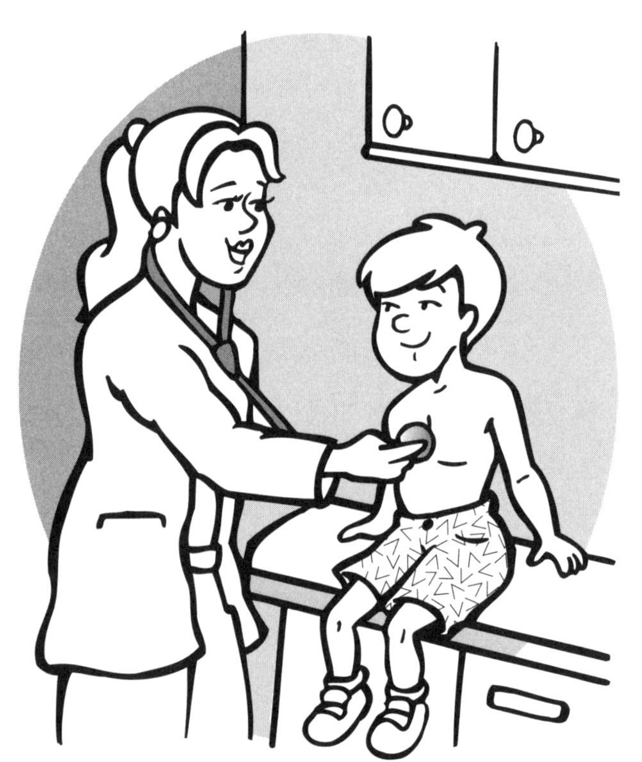

- ***Who*** is with the boy?
- ***What*** is the doctor doing?
- ***Where*** is the boy?
- ***When*** will the boy go home?
- ***Why*** did the boy visit the doctor?
- ***How*** does the boy feel?

Cut on dotted line

Florist

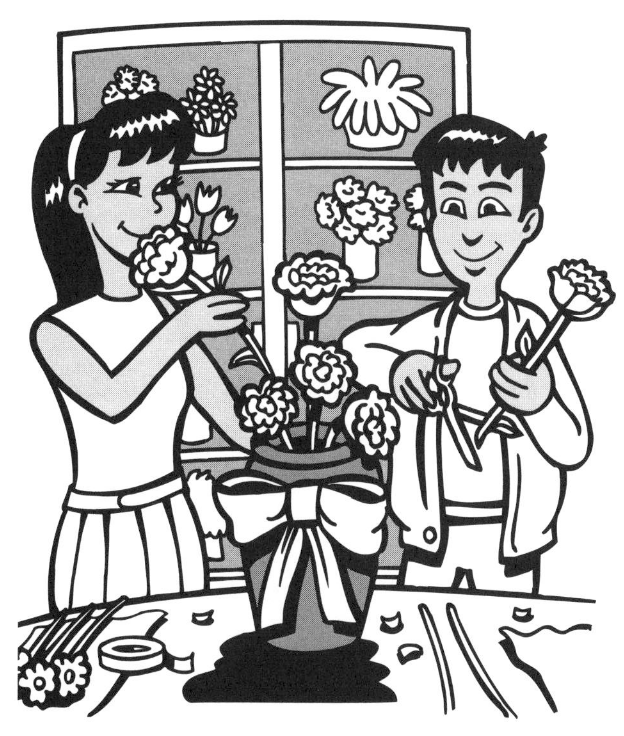

- ***Who*** is cutting the flowers?
- ***What*** is in the vase?

- ***Where*** do florists keep flowers?
- ***When*** do people send flowers?

- ***Why*** do florists keep flowers in a refrigerator?
- ***How*** do florists make a flower arrangement?

Cut on dotted line

Judge

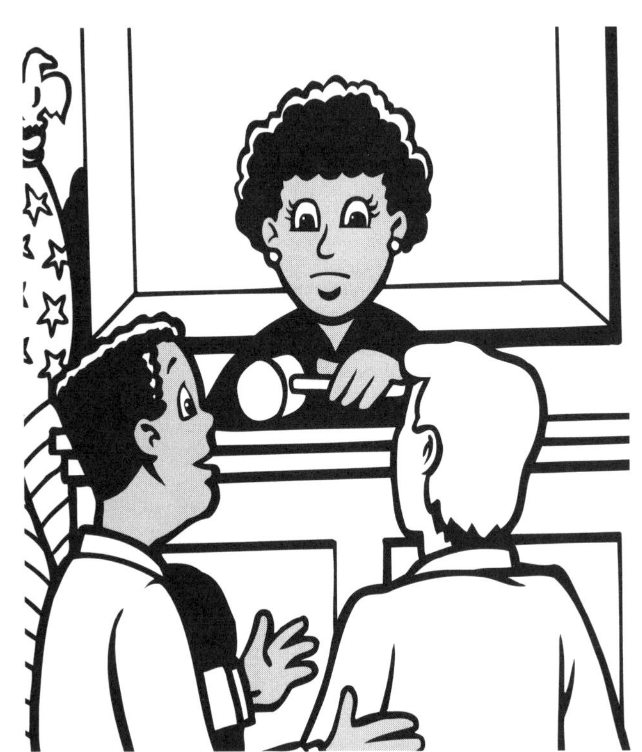

- ***Who*** is behind the bench?
- ***What*** is in the judge's hand?
- ***Where*** are these people?
- ***When*** do people go to court?
- ***Why*** does the judge have a gavel?
- ***How*** do people speak to a judge?

Cut on dotted line

Lawyer

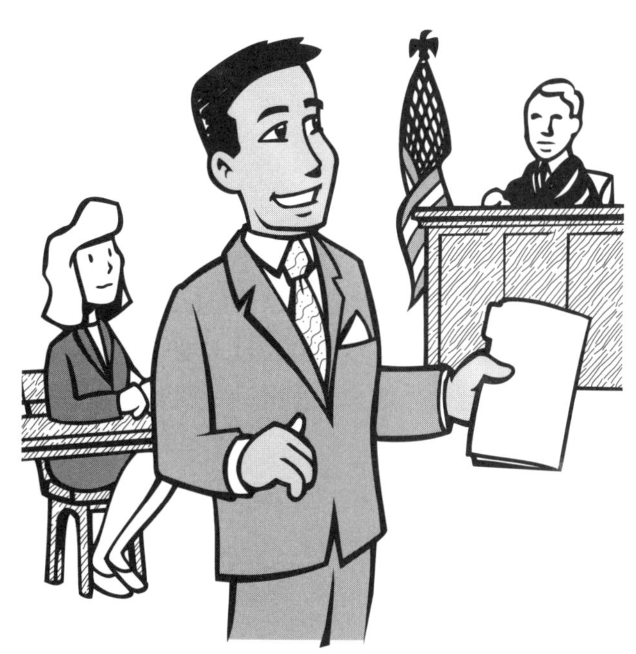

- ***Who*** helps people speak to a judge?
- ***What*** is the lawyer saying to the judge?

- ***Where*** do lawyers work?
- ***When*** do people need lawyers?

- ***Why*** is the lawyer standing?
- ***How*** does a lawyer help people?

Librarian

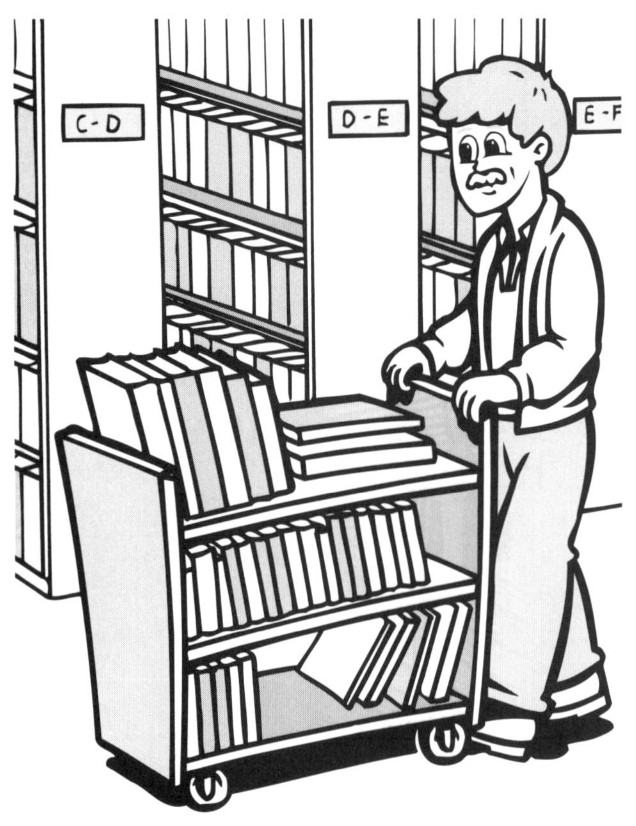

1 2 3 4

- ***Who*** is pushing the cart?
- ***What*** is in the cart?

- ***Where*** does this person work?
- ***When*** do books need to be put back on a shelf?

- ***Why*** does the librarian use a cart?
- ***How*** does the librarian know where to put the books on the shelf?

Cut on dotted line

Lifeguard

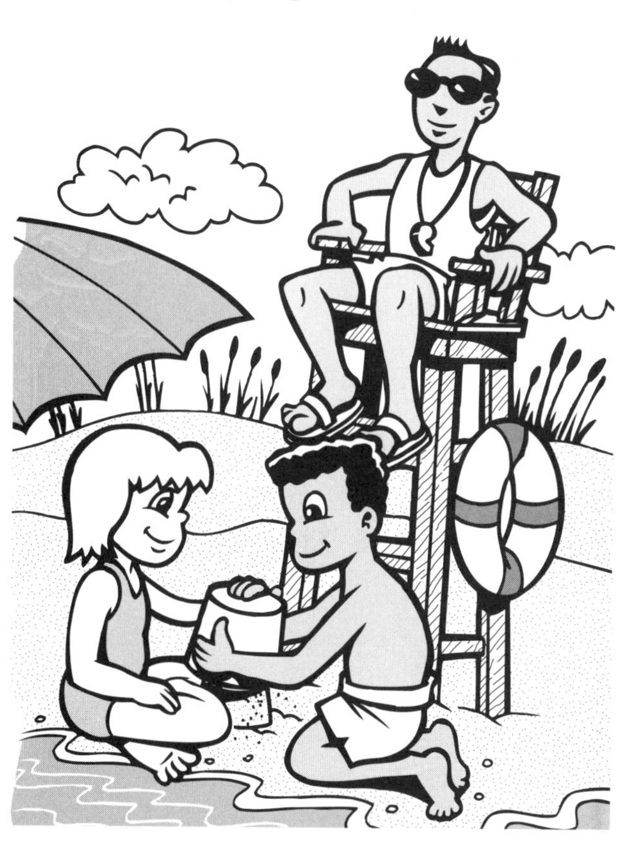

- **_Who_** is in the chair?
- **_What_** is the lifeguard wearing?
- **_Where_** do lifeguards work?
- **_When_** does a lifeguard jump down into the water?
- **_Why_** does a lifeguard blow his whistle?
- **_How_** do lifeguards save people?

1 2 3 4

Cut on dotted line

Magician

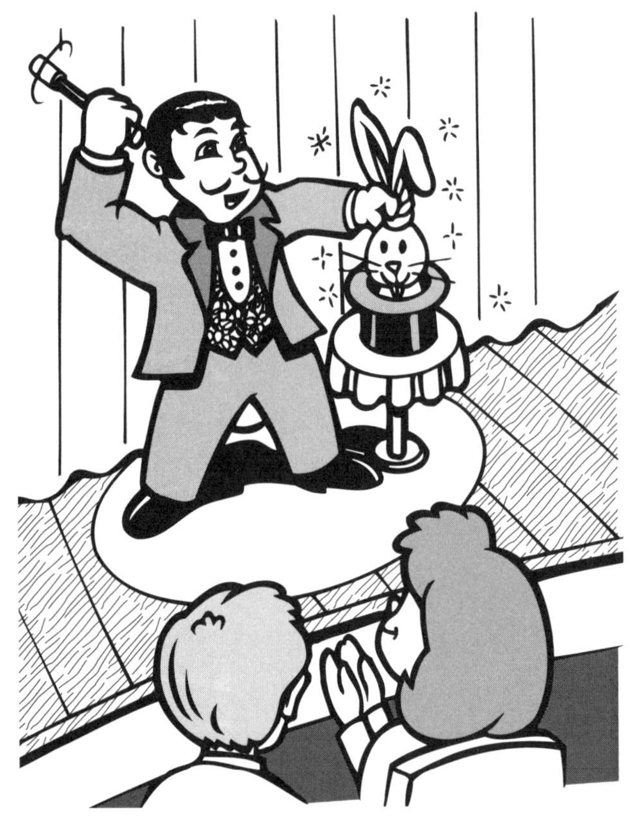

- ***Who*** is on the stage?
- ***What*** is the magician holding?

- ***Where*** did the rabbit come from?
- ***When*** does a magician say abracadabra?

- ***Why*** is the magician doing magic tricks?
- ***How*** does a magician know the audience likes his tricks?

Cut on dotted line

- ***When*** do people clean up?

- ***What*** is the man cleaning?

- ***Where*** is the water?

- ***Who*** is washing the floor?

2 3
1 4

Maids

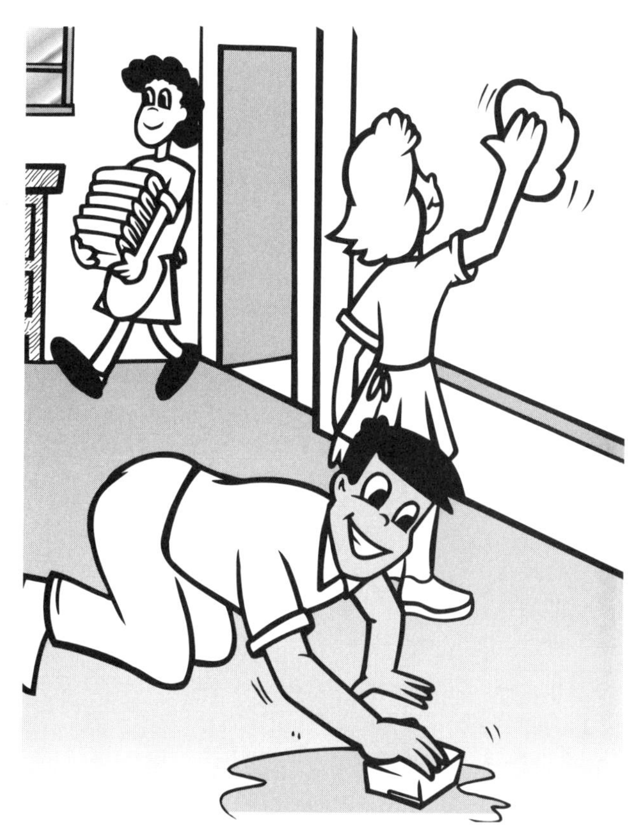

- ***Why*** do we use soap to clean things?

- ***How*** do you clean windows?

Pilot

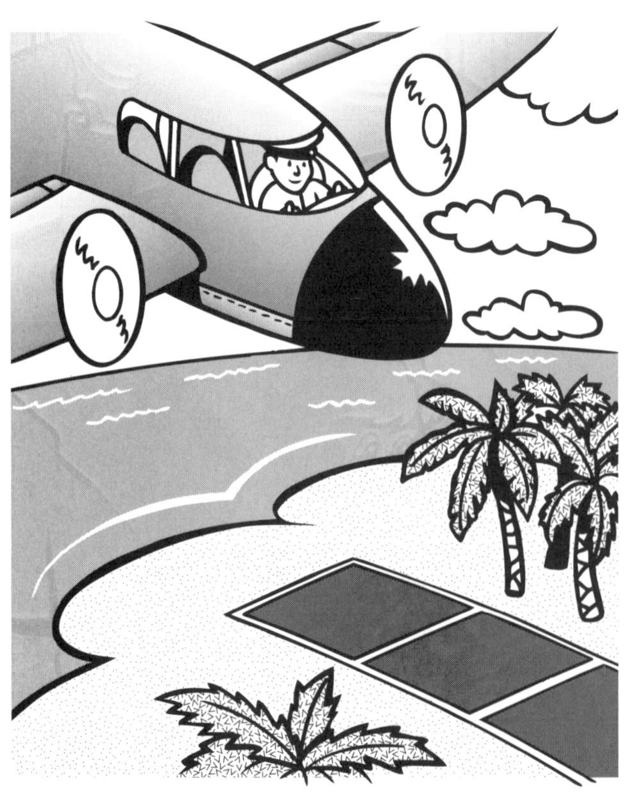

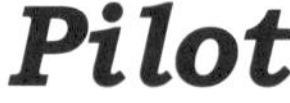

- ***Who*** flies an airplane?
- ***What*** are on the sides of an airplane?

- ***Where*** is the plane going?
- ***When*** do people ride in an airplane?

- ***Why*** are runways long?
- ***How*** does an airplane take off?

Cut on dotted line

Pirate

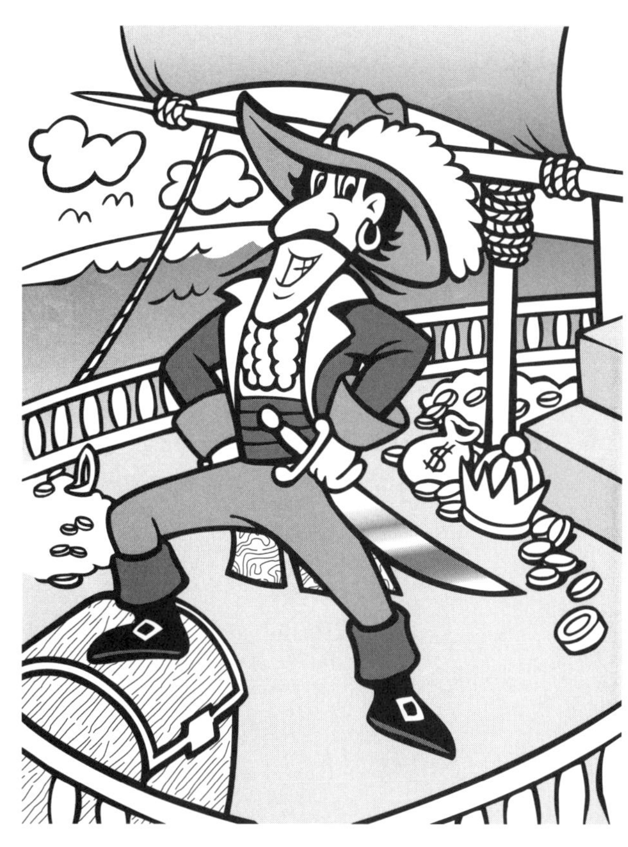

- ***Who*** is on the ship?
- ***What*** does he have?

- ***Where*** is the treasure?
- ***When*** will he spend his treasure?

1 2 3 4

- ***Why*** is the pirate happy?

- ***How*** does a pirate get lots of treasures?

Plumber

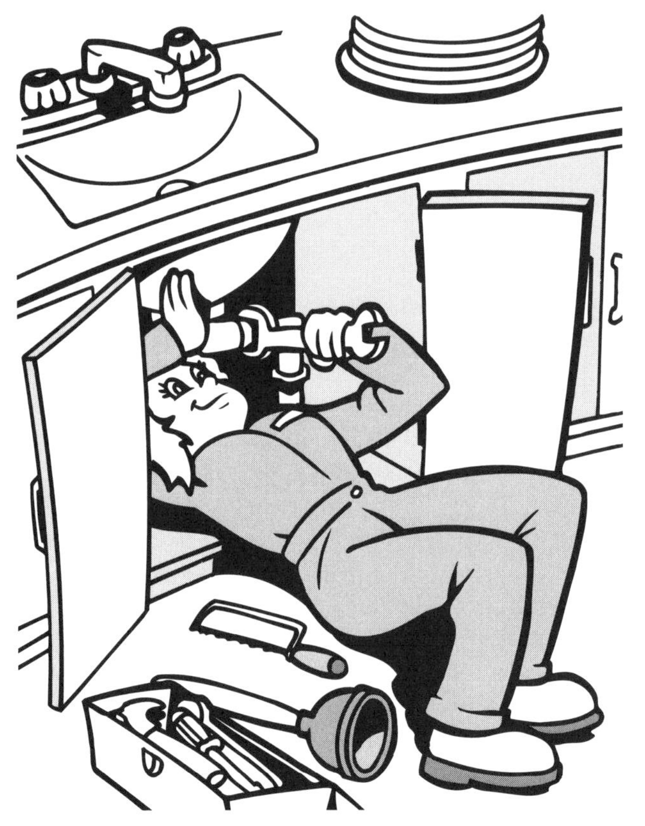

- ***Who*** is working on the pipes?
- ***What*** is plumber the checking?
- ***Where*** is the plumber?
- ***When*** does a plumber fix water pipes?
- ***Why*** do plumbers need tools?
- ***How*** do you know if a sink is clogged?

1 2 3 4

Cut on dotted line

Cut on dotted line

- ***What*** is the police officer wearing?
- ***Who*** writes speeding tickets?

- ***When*** does a police officer write a ticket?
- ***Where*** is the man?

2 3
1 4

Police Officer

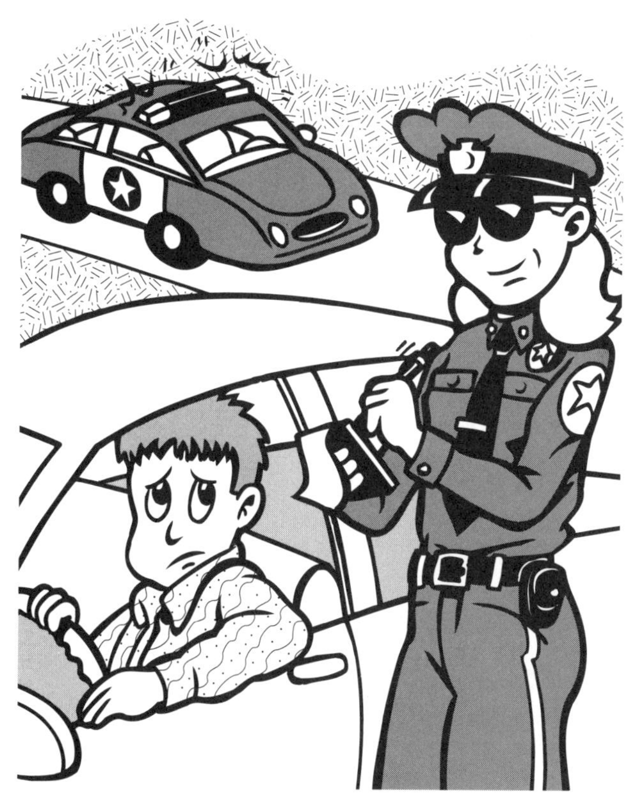

- ***Why*** do we have laws?
- ***How*** does the man in the car feel?

President

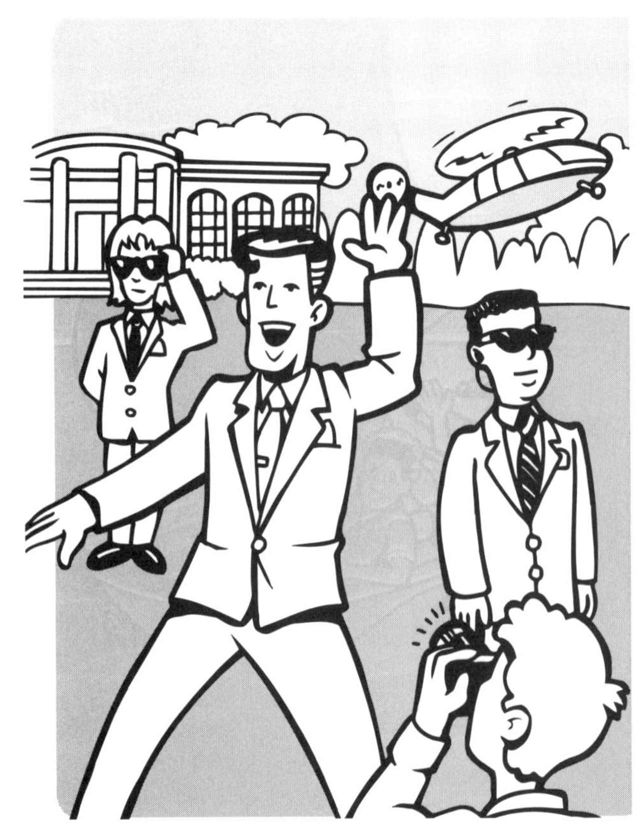

- ***Who*** lives in the big white house?
- ***What*** is landing on the lawn?

- ***Where*** does the president live?
- ***When*** do secret service agents go with the president?

- ***Why*** does the president have a helicopter?
- ***How*** would you become president?

1 2 3 4

Cut on dotted line

Railroad Engineer

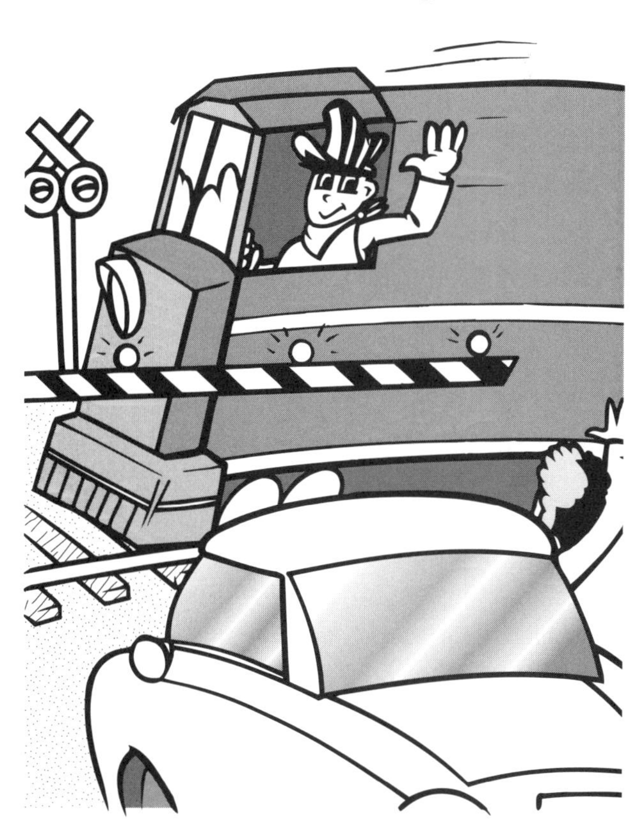

- ***Who*** drives a train?

- ***What*** does the train travel on?

- ***Where*** is the train engineer?

- ***When*** does a train blow its whistle?

- ***Why*** are the cars stopped for the train?

- ***How*** do you know when a train is coming?

Cut on dotted line

Occupations

Ranger

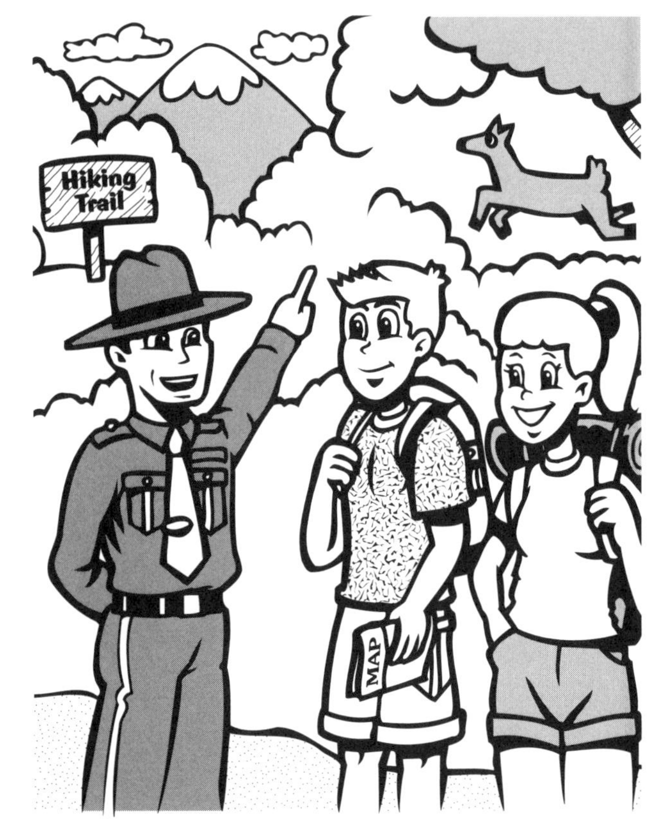

1

- ***Who*** are the hikers talking with?

- ***What*** is in the woods?

2

- ***Where*** does a forest ranger work?

- ***When*** do you need a forest ranger?

3

- ***Why*** do the hikers need the ranger's help?

- ***How*** do you find your way in the woods?

4

Cut on dotted line

1

Scientist

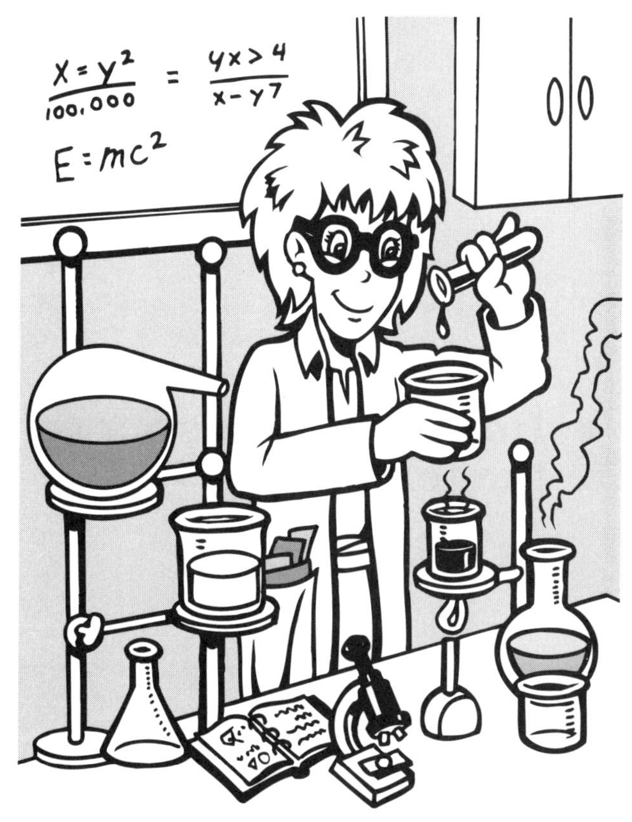

2

- ***Who*** is doing the science experiments?
- ***What*** is she making?

3

- ***Where*** is she working?
- ***When*** will her experiment be over?

4

- ***Why*** is she wearing goggles?
- ***How*** do you invent something new?

Cut on dotted line

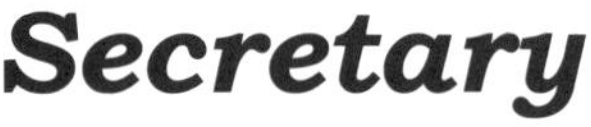

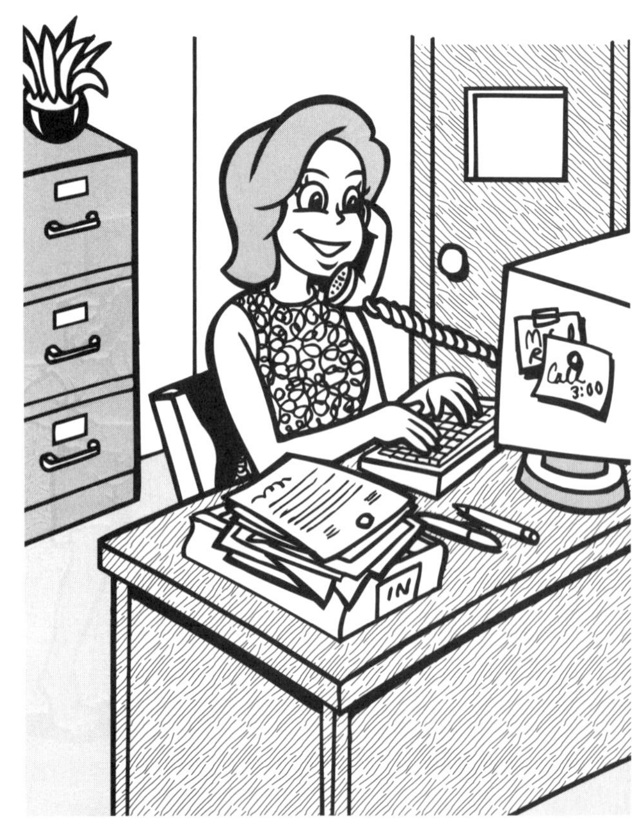

- ***Who*** is typing?
- ***What*** does she have next to her ear?

- ***Where*** is she sitting?
- ***When*** will she go home?

- ***Why*** is she so busy?
- ***How*** do you answer the telephone?

1 2 3 4

Cut on dotted line

Speech-Language Pathologist

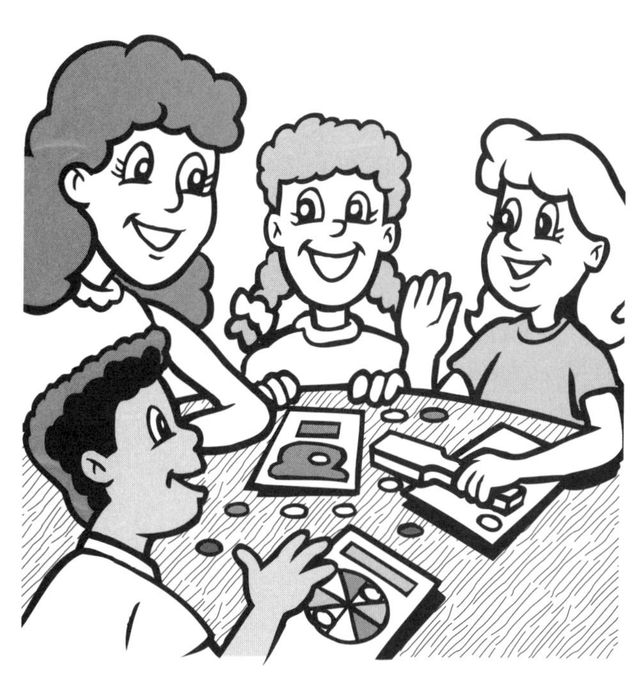

- ***Who*** is working with the children?

- ***What*** do children do in speech therapy?

- ***Where*** are the children?

- ***When*** does a child go to speech therapy?

- ***Why*** is speech and language important?

- ***How*** are a speech therapist and a teacher alike?

1 2 3 4

Supermarket Cashier

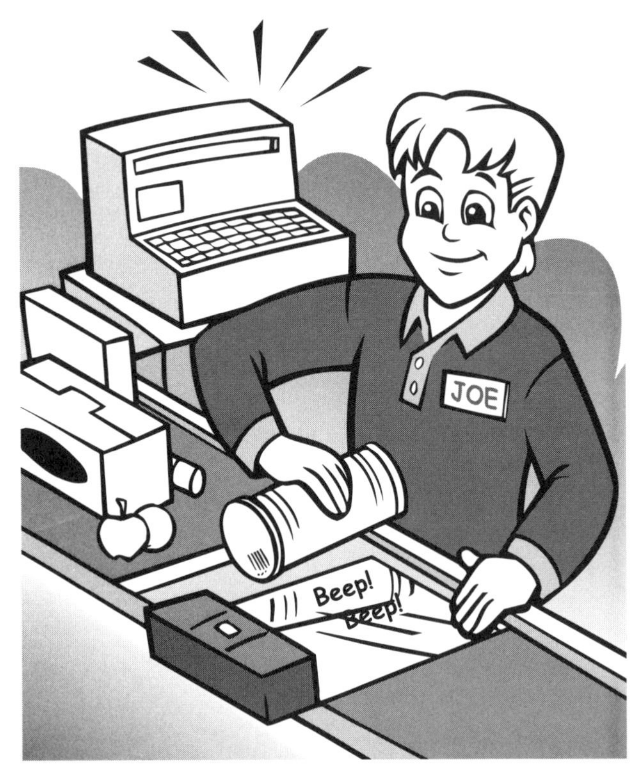

- ***Who*** collects the money at the grocery store?

- ***What*** is the man wearing?

- ***Where*** is the money kept?

- ***When*** does the man collect the money?

- ***Why*** do people go to a grocery store?

- ***How*** do you know the cost of each item?

1 2 3 4

Cut on dotted line

Cut on dotted line

Teacher

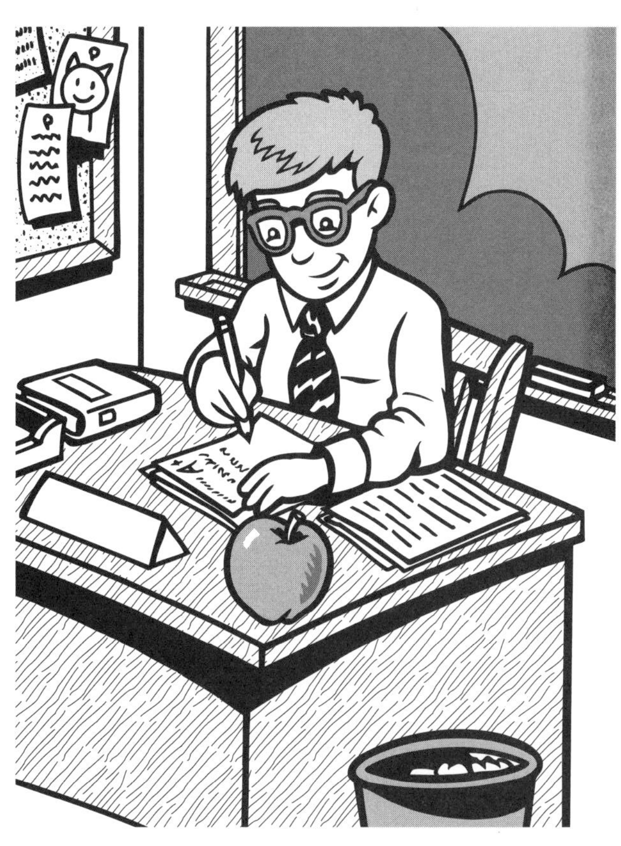

- ***Who*** is grading the test?
- ***What*** does he have on his desk?
- ***When*** do you do your homework?
- ***Where*** is he sitting?

1 2 3 4

- ***Why*** does a teacher grade papers?
- ***How*** do you study for your tests?

- ***What*** does she use to steer the truck?

- ***When*** will she pull off the road?

- ***Who*** is driving the truck?

- ***Where*** is she sitting?

1 2 3 4

Truck Driver

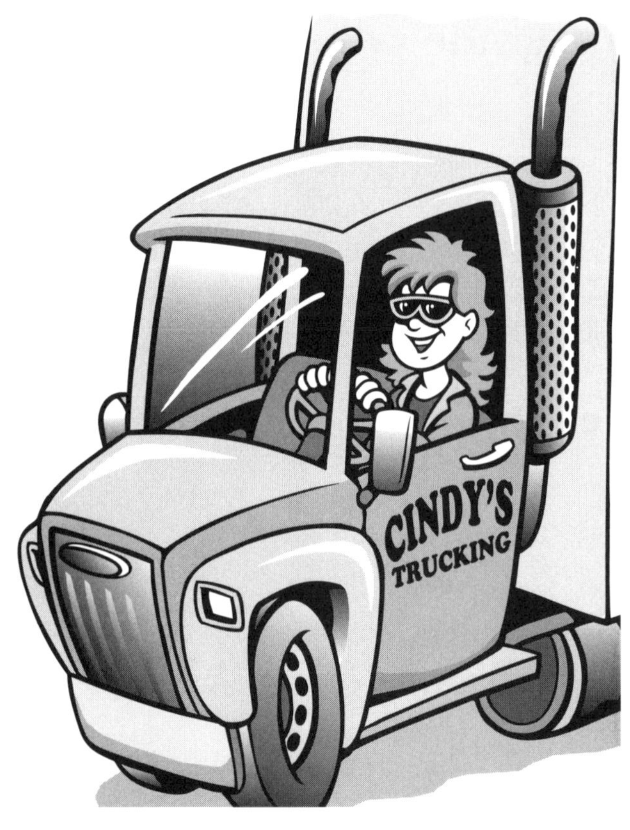

- ***Why*** are trucks so big?

- ***How*** did the lady learn to drive the truck?

Cut on dotted line

Waitress

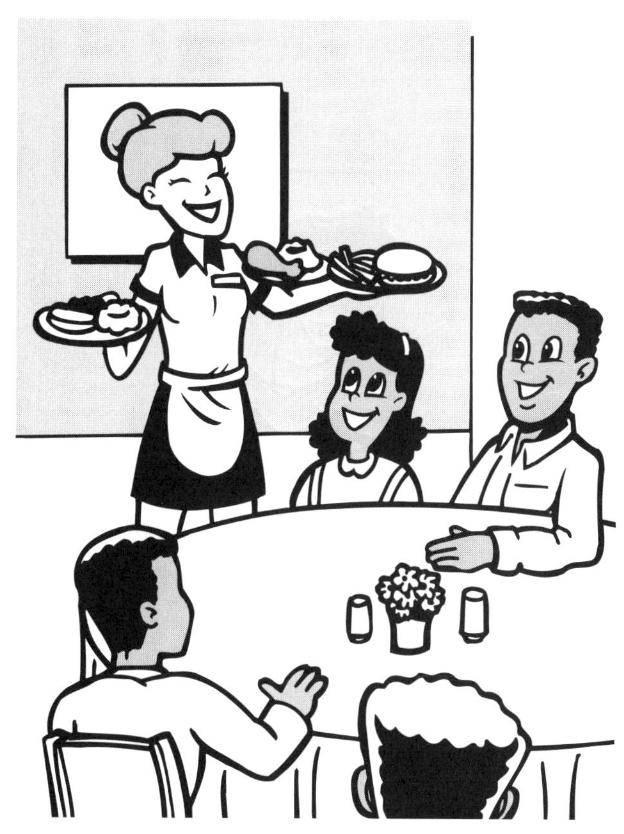

1 2 3 4

- **Who** serves food at a restaurant?
- **What** is she carrying?

- **Where** did the waitress get the food?
- **When** do you go out to eat?

- ***Why*** is she carrying so much food?
- ***How*** do you order food at a restaurant?

Cut on dotted line

Zoo Keeper

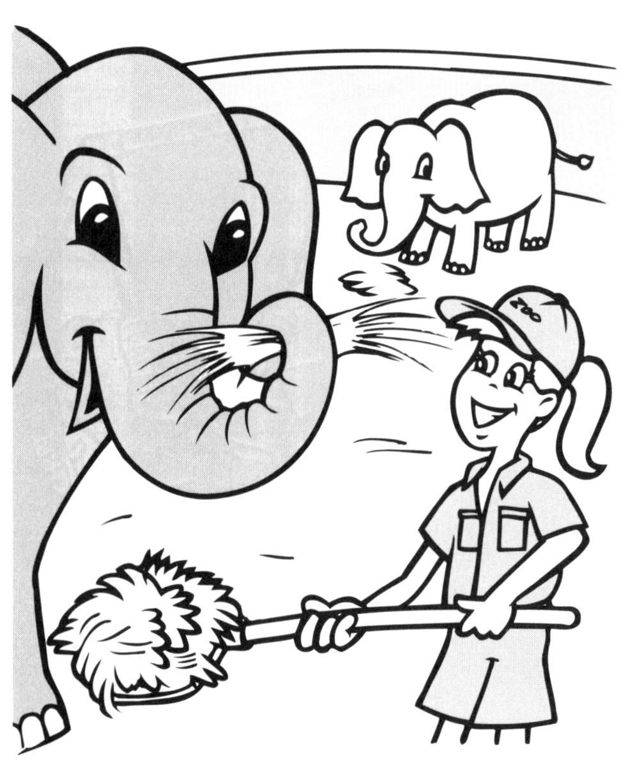

- ***Who*** feeds the zoo animals?

- ***What*** do elephants eat?

- ***Where*** is the elephant's mouth?

- ***When*** does the zookeeper clean up at the zoo?

- ***Why*** are these elephants happy?

- ***How*** does an elephant drink water?

Cut on dotted line

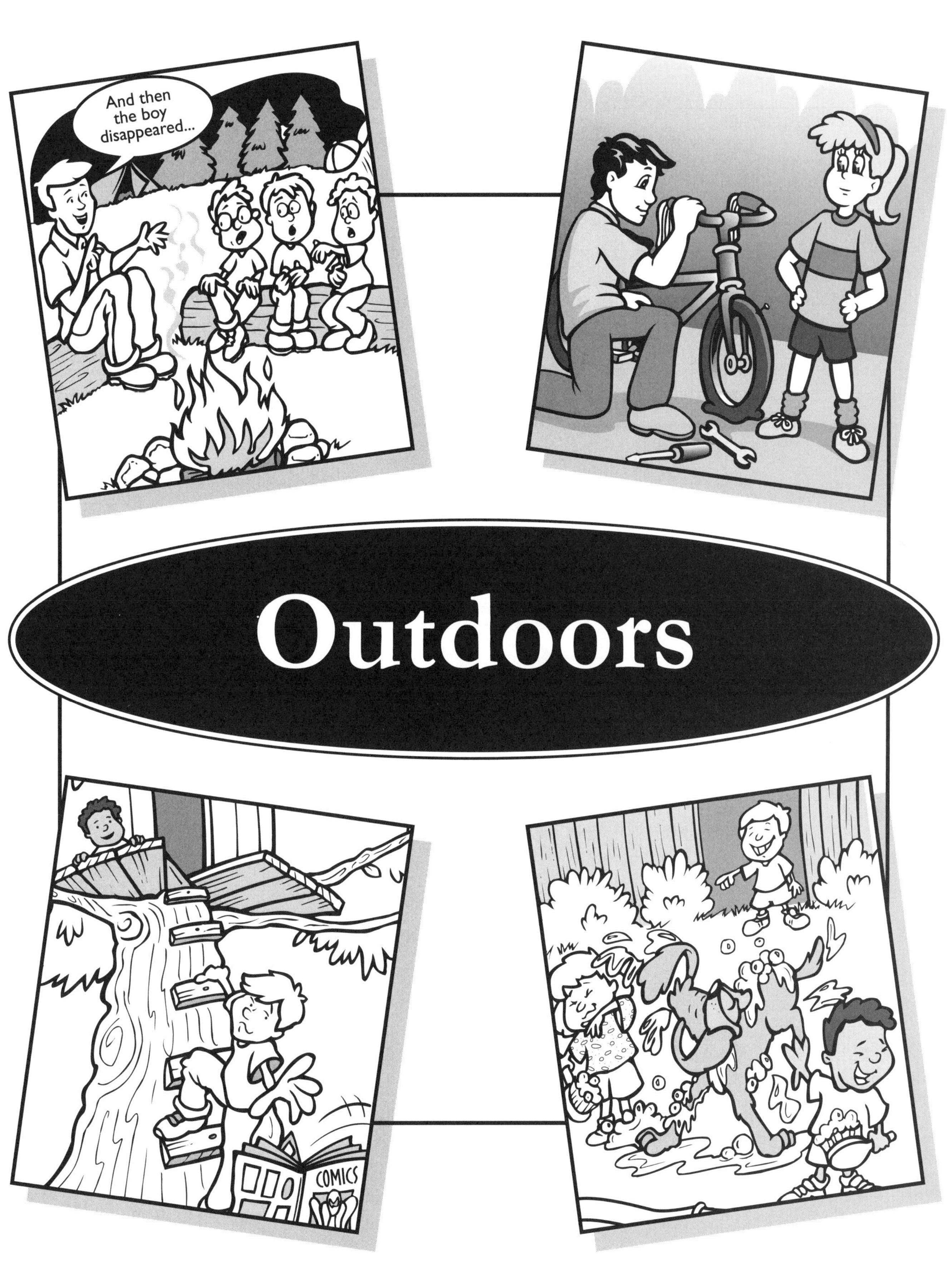
And then the boy disappeared...
Outdoors
COMICS

Birdbath

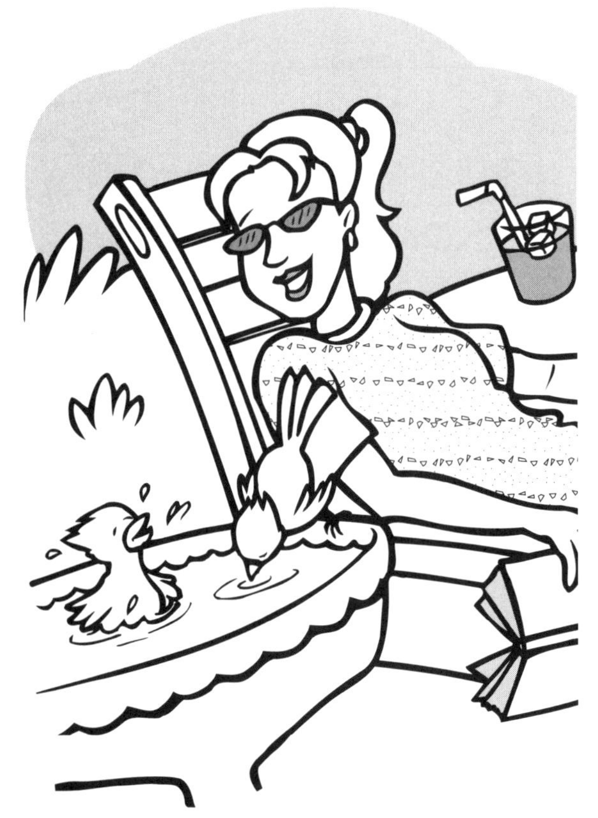

- ***Who*** is watching the birds?

- ***What*** are the birds in?

- ***Where*** is the birdbath?

- ***When*** do birds take a bath?

- ***Why*** are the birds happy?

- ***How*** do you take a bath?

Cut on dotted line

Campfire

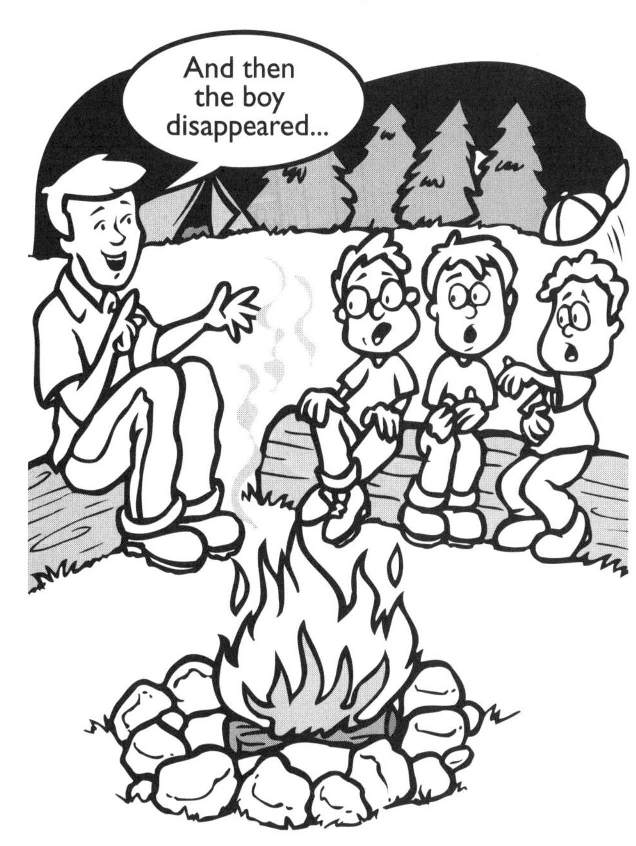

- ***Who*** is telling a story?
- ***What*** are the children sitting around?

- ***Where*** is the smoke going?
- ***When*** do people have campfires?

- ***Why*** do the children look frightened?
- ***How*** do you build a campfire?

1 2 3 4

Climbing the Tree

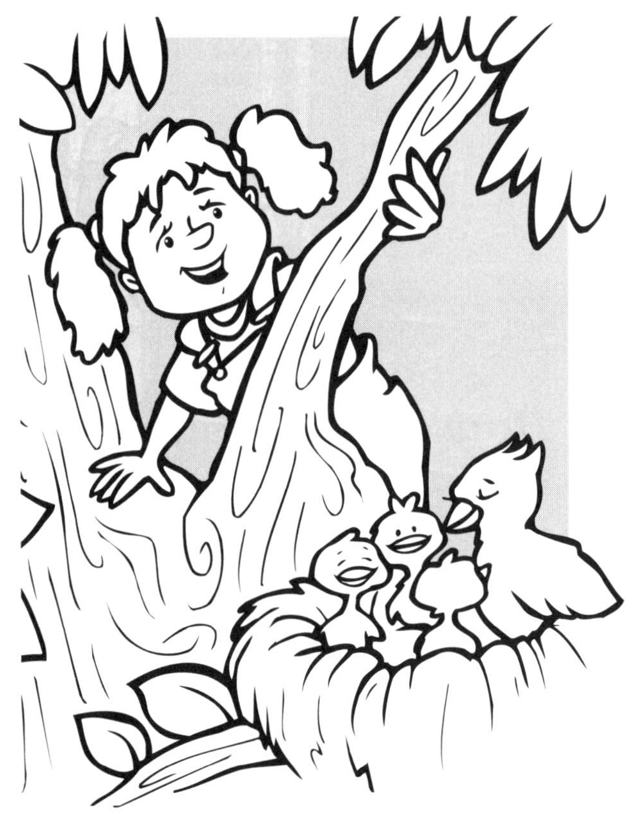

- ***Who*** is climbing the tree?
- ***What*** else is in the tree?

- ***Where*** is the girl climbing?
- ***When*** will she come down from the tree?

- ***Why*** should the girl be careful?
- ***How*** do you climb a tree?

Mowing the Lawn

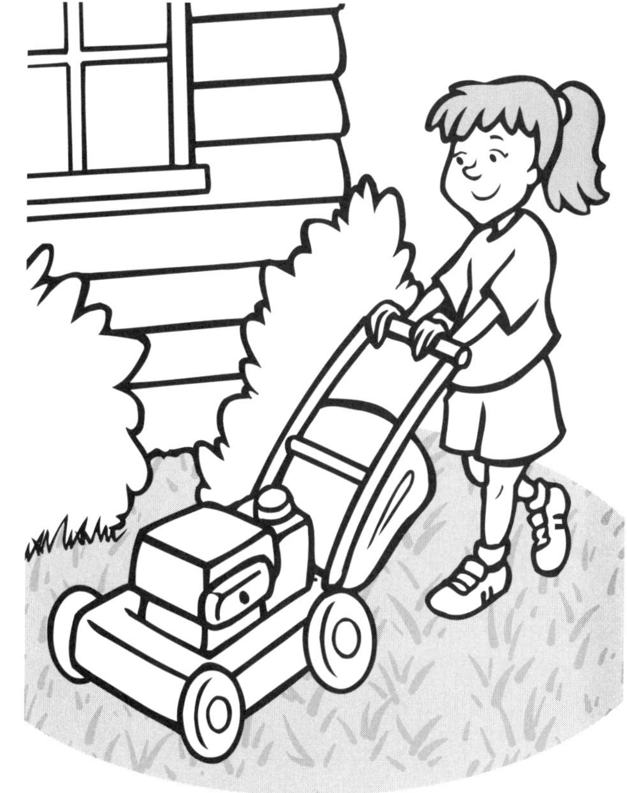

- ***Who*** is mowing the lawn?
- ***What*** does the lady use to mow the lawn?

- ***Where*** is she mowing?
- ***When*** do people mow their lawns?

- ***Why*** do people need to mow their lawns?
- ***How*** do you start a lawn mower?

- ***What*** is on the ground?

- ***When*** do people eat apples?

- ***Who*** is running under the trees?

- ***Where*** is the boy eating the apple?

Orchard

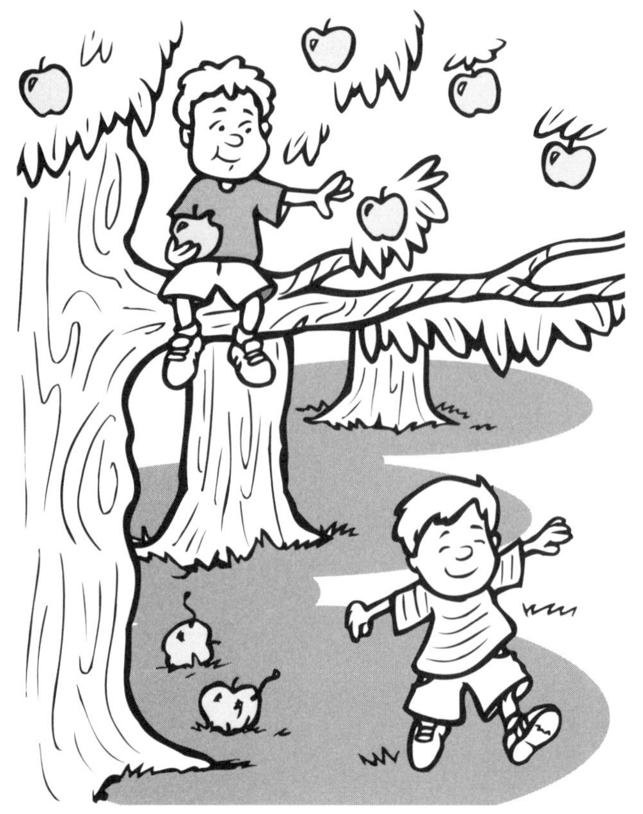

- ***Why*** did some apples fall to the ground?

- ***How*** do you eat an apple?

Cut on dotted line

Cut on dotted line

Picnic

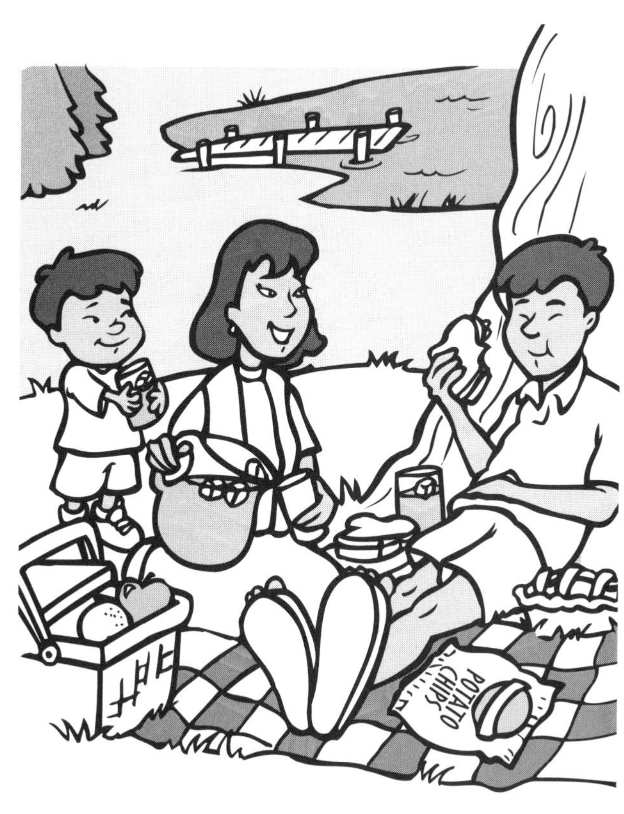

- ***Who*** is eating the sandwich?
- ***What*** are the people drinking?

- ***Where*** are they eating?
- ***When*** do people go on a picnic?

- ***Why*** are they sitting on a blanket?
- ***How*** do you pack a picnic lunch?

Repairing a Bike

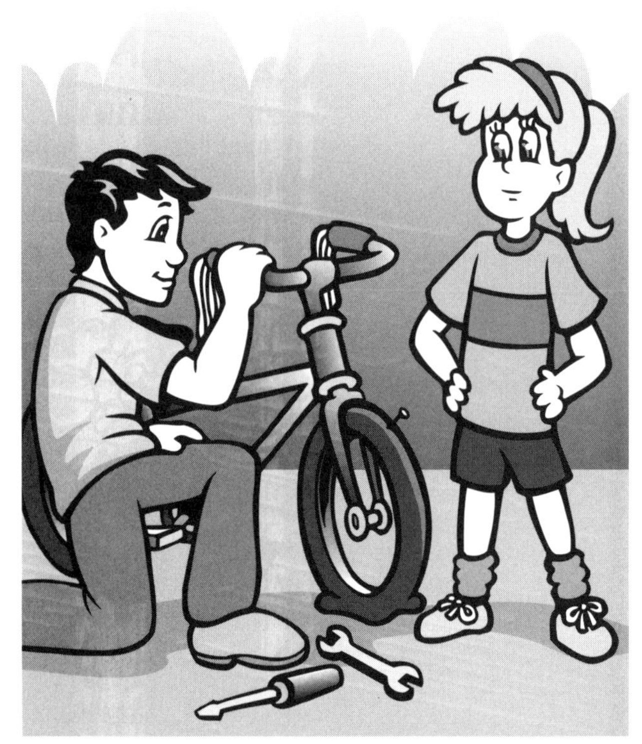

- ***Who*** is fixing the tire?
- ***What*** made the tire go flat?

- ***Where*** are the man and the girl?
- ***When*** will the girl ride her bike again?

- ***Why*** do you need to fix a flat tire?
- ***How*** do you fix a flat tire?

1 2 3 4

Cut on dotted line

Seed Planting

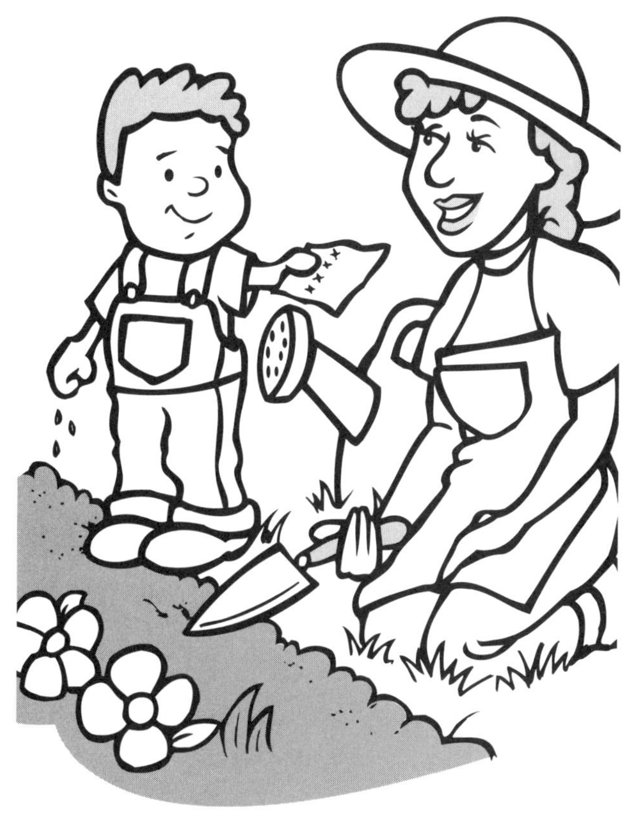

- ***Who*** is in the garden?
- ***What*** are they planting?

- ***Where*** is the watering can?
- ***When*** do people plant a garden?

- ***Why*** do seeds need water?
- ***How*** do you make a garden grow?

Cut on dotted line

Treehouse

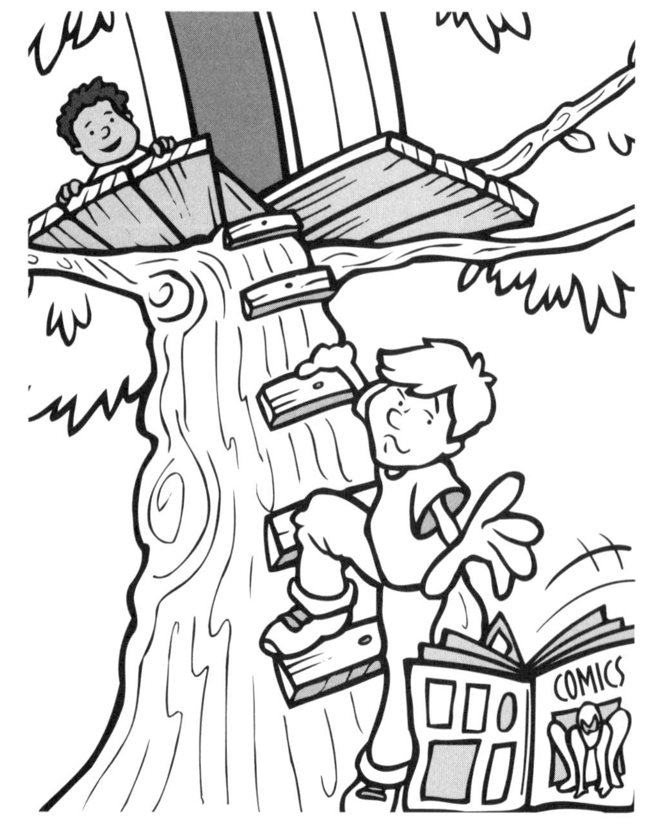

- ***Who*** is climbing the ladder?
- ***What*** did the boy drop?

- ***Where*** is this treehouse?
- ***When*** will the boys go back home?

- ***Why*** is the treehouse up so high?
- ***How*** do you build a treehouse?

Cut on dotted line

1 2 3 4

Washing the Car

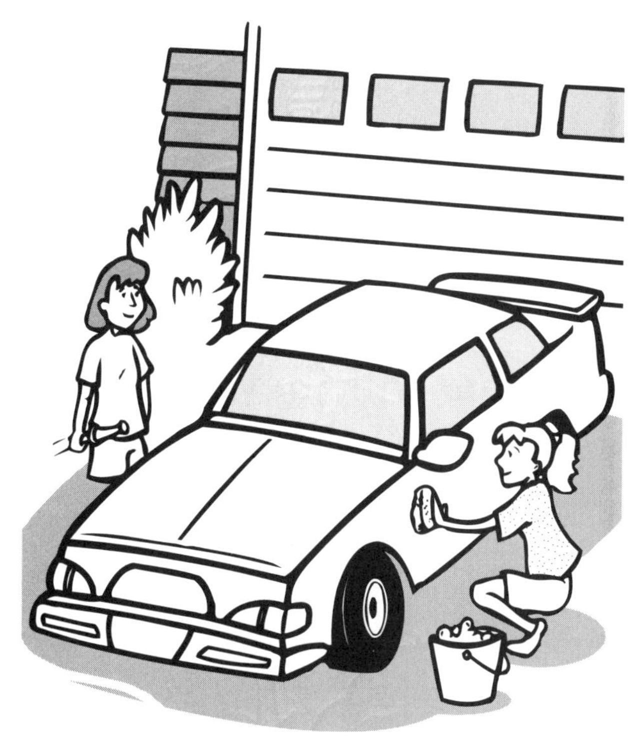

- ***Why*** does a car need to be washed?

- ***How*** does a car get dirty?

- ***Who*** is holding the hose?

- ***What*** do you use to wash a car?

- ***Where*** is the car?

- ***When*** do you rinse the car?

Washing the Dog

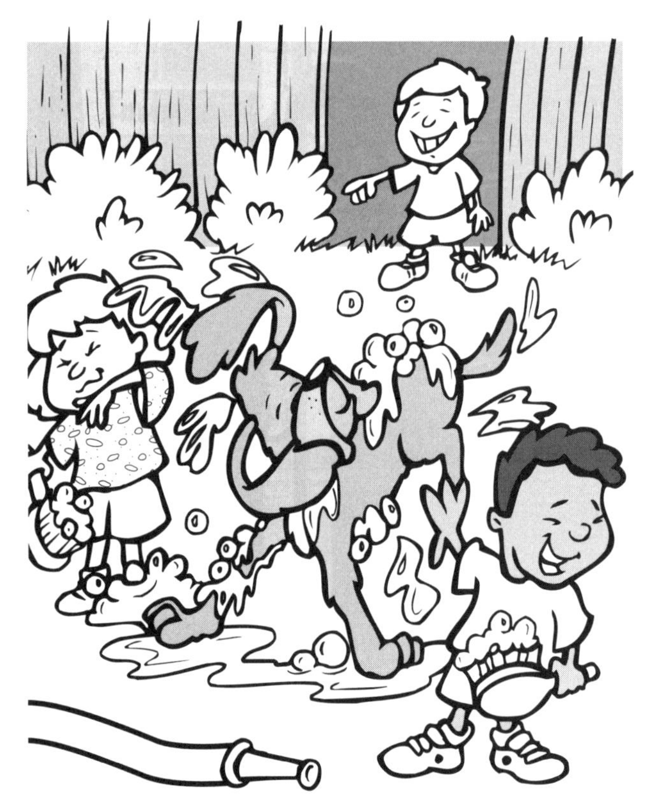

- ***Who*** is washing the dog?
- ***What*** do the children have in their hands?

- ***Where*** is the hose?
- ***When*** do you wash a dog?

- ***Why*** is the other boy laughing?
- ***How*** will they get the soap off the dog?

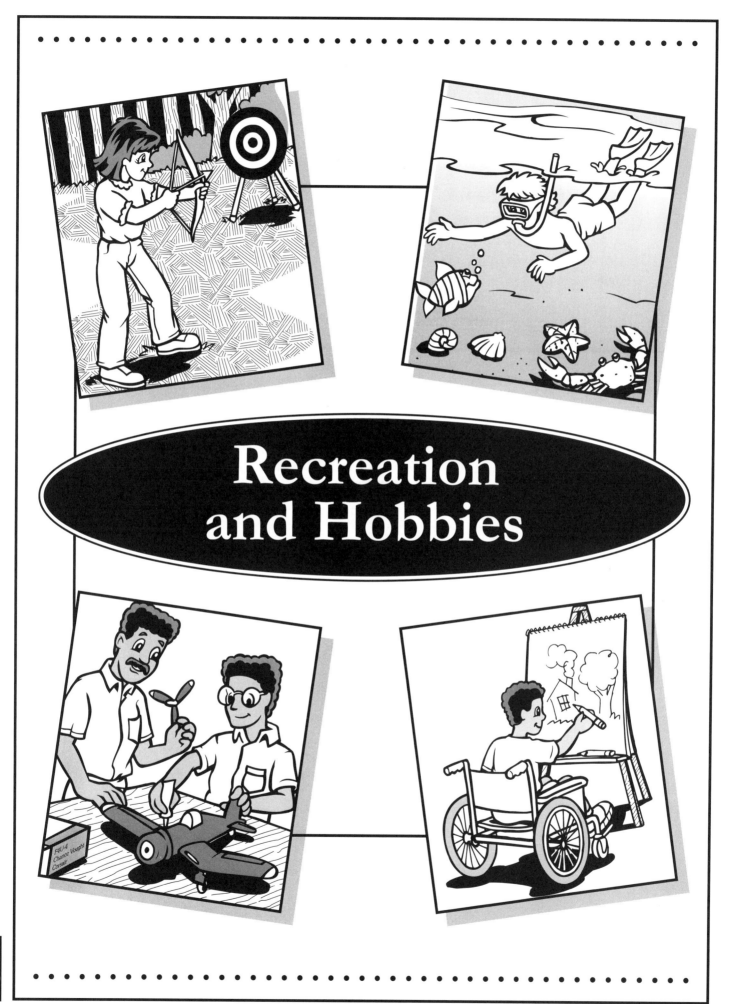
Recreation
and Hobbies
F4U-4
Chance Vought
Corsair

Archery

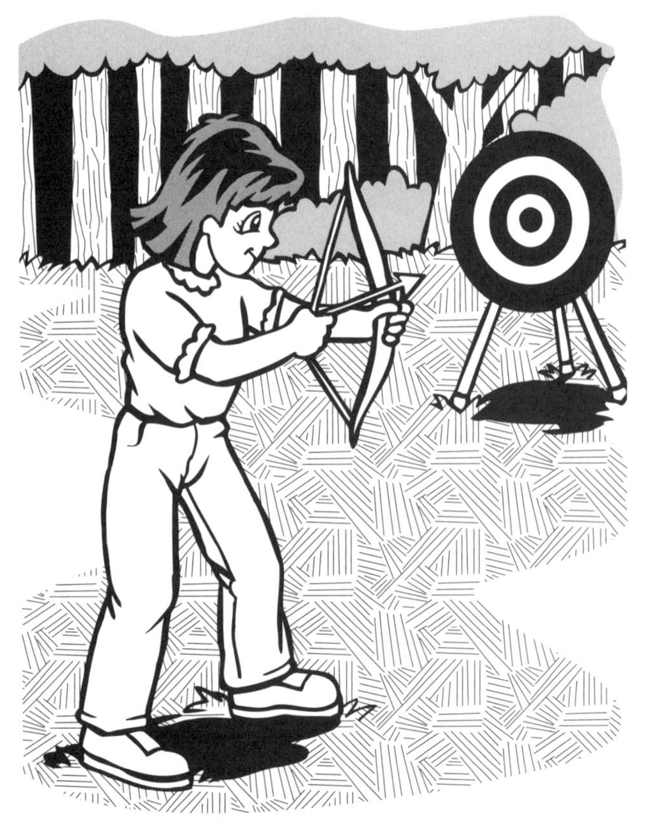

- ***Who*** uses a bow and arrow?
- ***What*** is the archer aiming for?

- ***Where*** should people shoot their arrows?
- ***When*** is it safe to walk near the archer?

- ***Why*** is this sport dangerous?
- ***How*** does a person shoot an arrow?

Cut on dotted line

Art Table

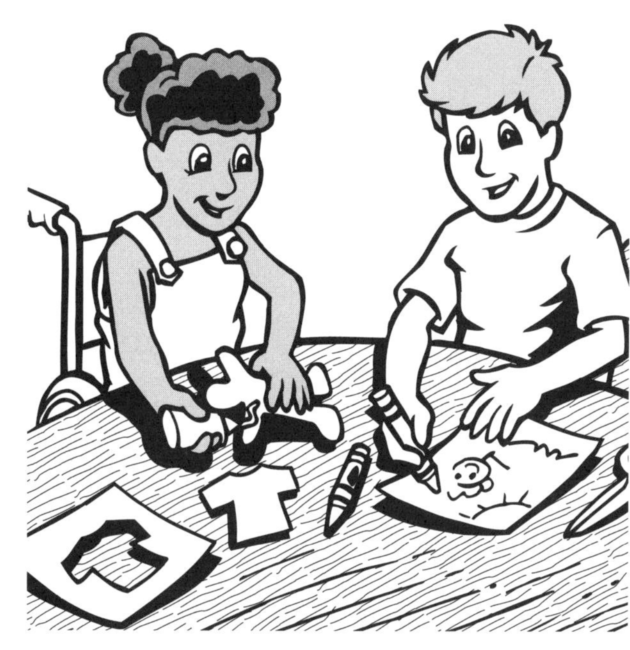

- ***Who*** is coloring at the table?
- ***What*** type of art projects do you like?
- ***Where*** are the crayons?
- ***When*** do you color a picture?

2 3

4 1

- ***Why*** are the scissors on the table?
- ***How*** do you glue pictures?

Cut on dotted line

Recreation and Hobbies

Cut on dotted line

1 2 3 4

Basketball

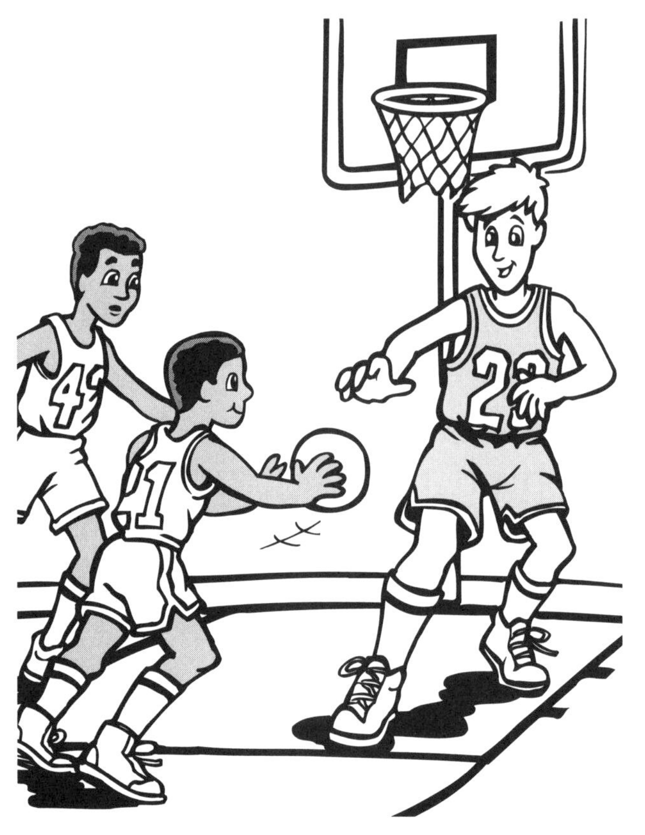

- ***Who*** has the ball?
- ***What*** are the boys wearing?

- ***Where*** do you play basketball?
- ***When*** do you pass the ball?

- ***Why*** do you throw the ball at the basket?
- ***How*** do you dribble the ball?

Bike Riding

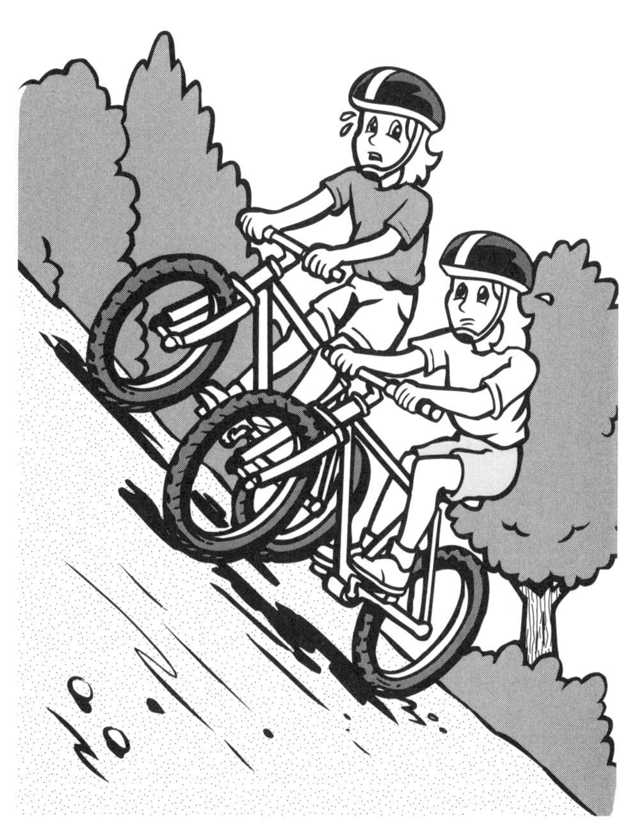

- ***Who*** is tired?
- ***What*** are the girls riding?
- ***Where*** are they?
- ***When*** do people ride a bike?
- ***Why*** do they look tired?
- ***How*** do you ride a bike?

1 2 3 4

Cut on dotted line

Building a Birdhouse

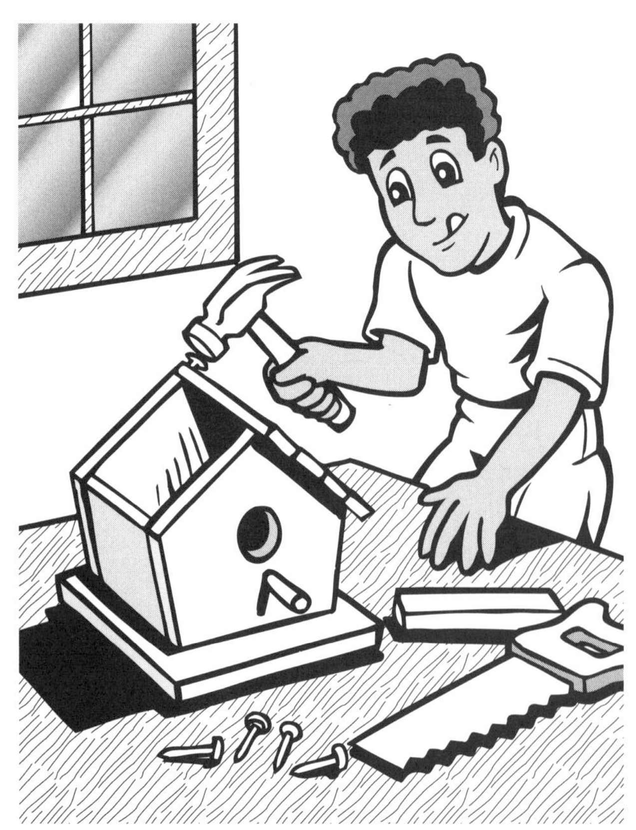

- ***Who*** is building the birdhouse?
- ***What*** is needed to make a birdhouse?
- ***When*** do birds use a birdhouse?
- ***Where*** should a birdhouse be placed?
- ***Why*** do people make birdhouses?
- ***How*** will the birds find the birdhouse?

1

Cake Decorating

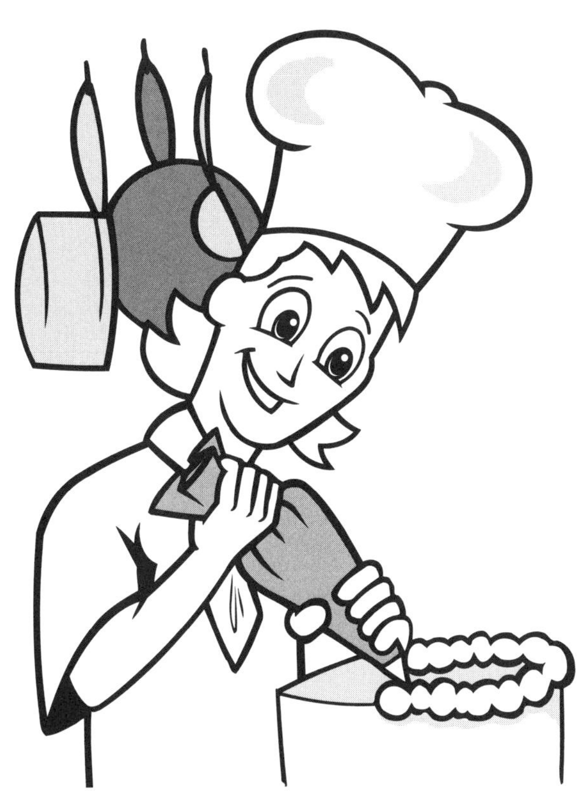

2

- ***Who*** makes cakes?
- ***What*** goes on top of a cake?

3

- ***Where*** does a cake bake?
- ***When*** do people make cakes?

4

- ***Why*** is the woman wearing a hat?
- ***How*** long does it take a cake to bake?

Carousel

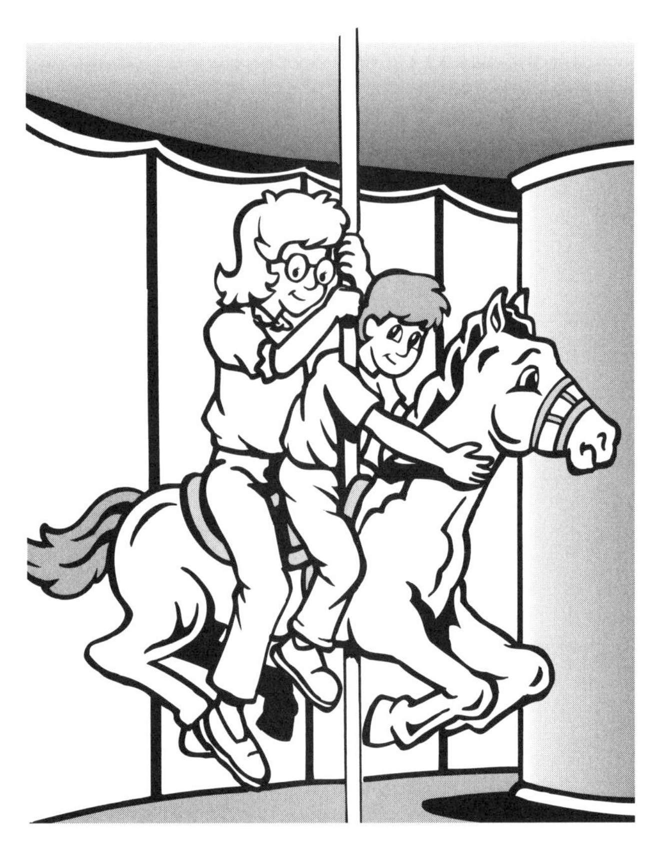

- ***Who*** is riding the carousel?
- ***What*** are they holding onto?
- ***When*** will they get down from the horse?
- ***Where*** are the people sitting?
- ***Why*** are they holding onto the pole?
- ***How*** will they feel when the carousel stops?

1 2 3 4

Cut on dotted line

Cut on dotted line

Checkers

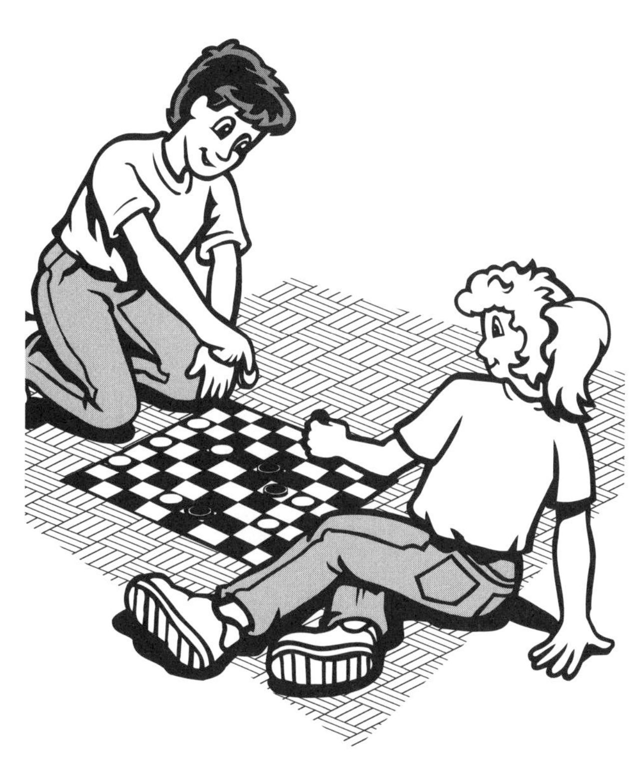

1 2 3 4

- ***Who*** is playing checkers?

- ***What*** are the children wearing?

- ***Where*** is a checker game kept?

- ***When*** will the children stop playing checkers?

- ***Why*** are they playing on the floor?

- ***How*** do you play checkers?

Choir

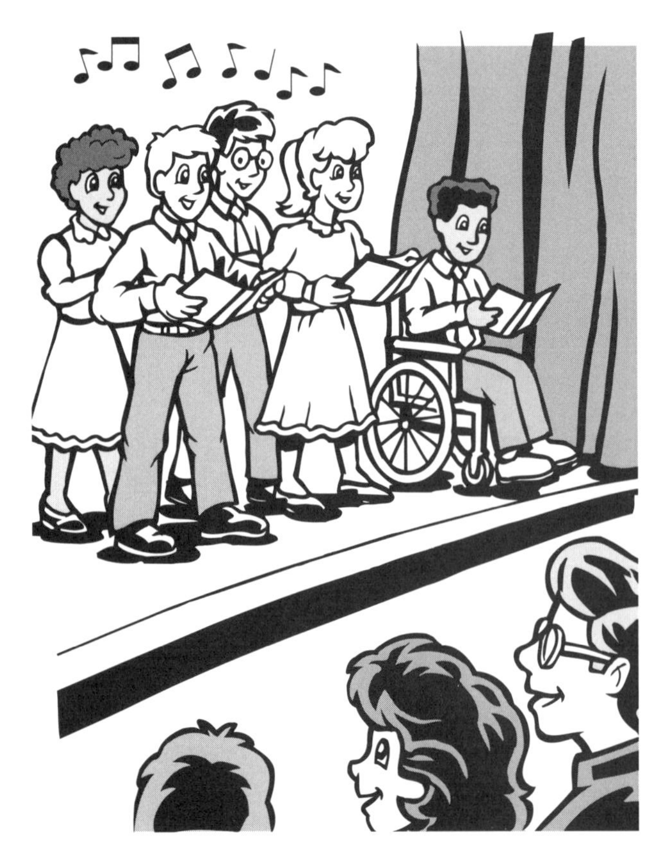

- ***Who*** is watching the choir?
- ***What*** are the children singing?

1 2 3 4

- ***Where*** is the choir?
- ***When*** do you sing?

- ***Why*** are the people smiling?
- ***How*** do you know the words to a song?

Cut on dotted line

Cut on dotted line

Clown

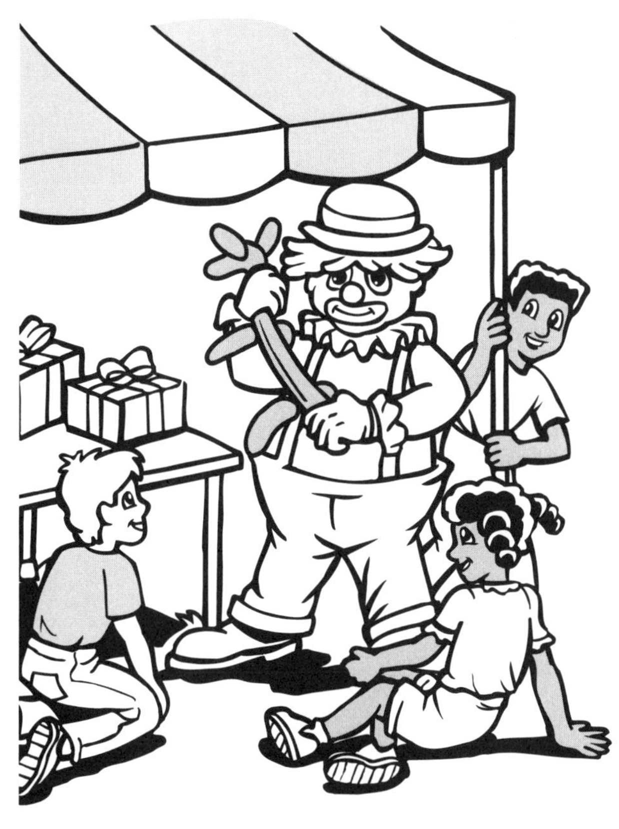

1 2 3 4

- ***Who*** is making the children laugh?
- ***What*** is the clown making?

- ***Where*** is the clown?
- ***When*** do people open presents?

- ***Why*** do clowns come to parties?
- ***How*** do you blow up a balloon?

Diving Board

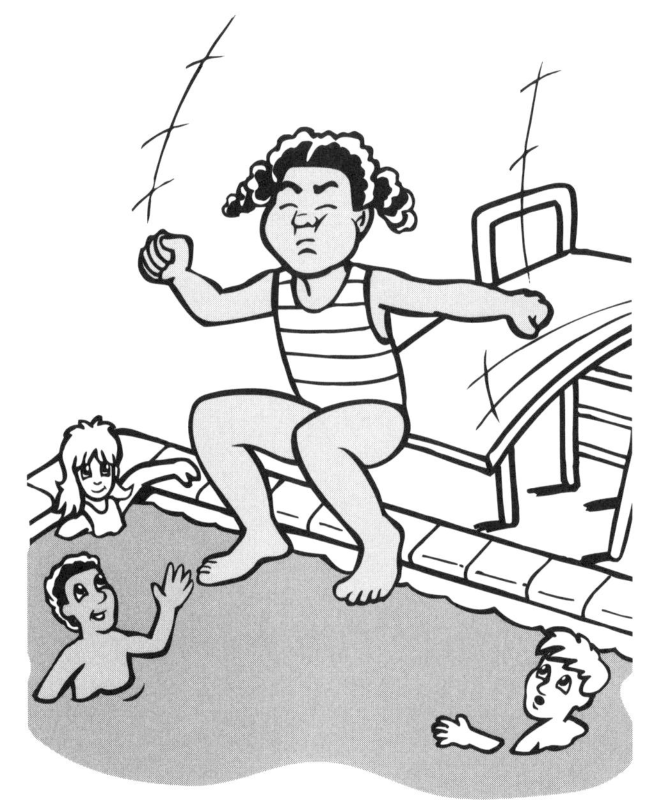

- ***Who*** is jumping?
- ***What*** is she jumping from?
- ***Where*** are the other children?
- ***When*** do people go to the pool?
- ***Why*** is she holding her breath?
- ***How*** do you make a big splash in the swimming pool?

Cut on dotted line

Drawing

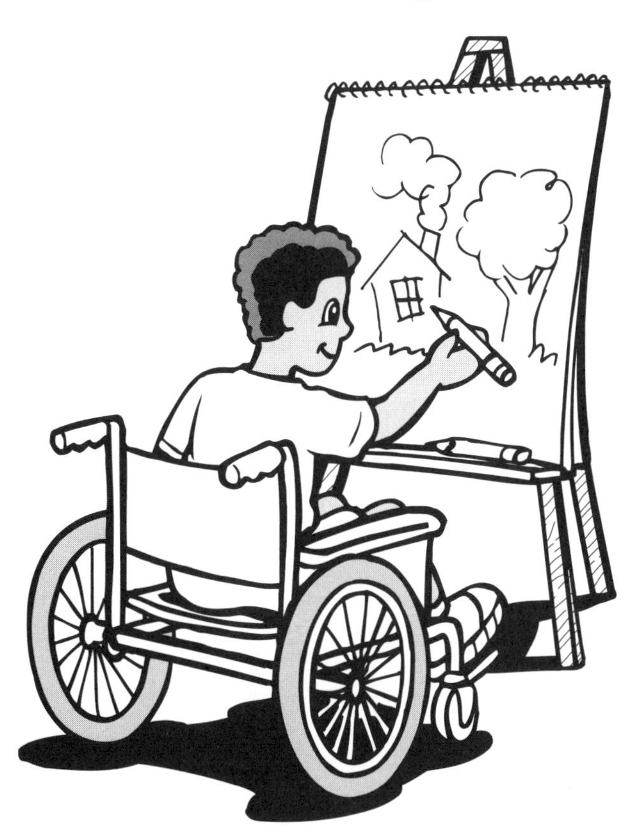

- ***Who*** is drawing the picture?
- ***What*** is needed to sketch a picture?
- ***Where*** is the boy drawing?
- ***When*** will he be finished?
- ***Why*** is he using the easel?
- ***How*** long does it take you to draw a cat?

Cut on dotted line

Fishing

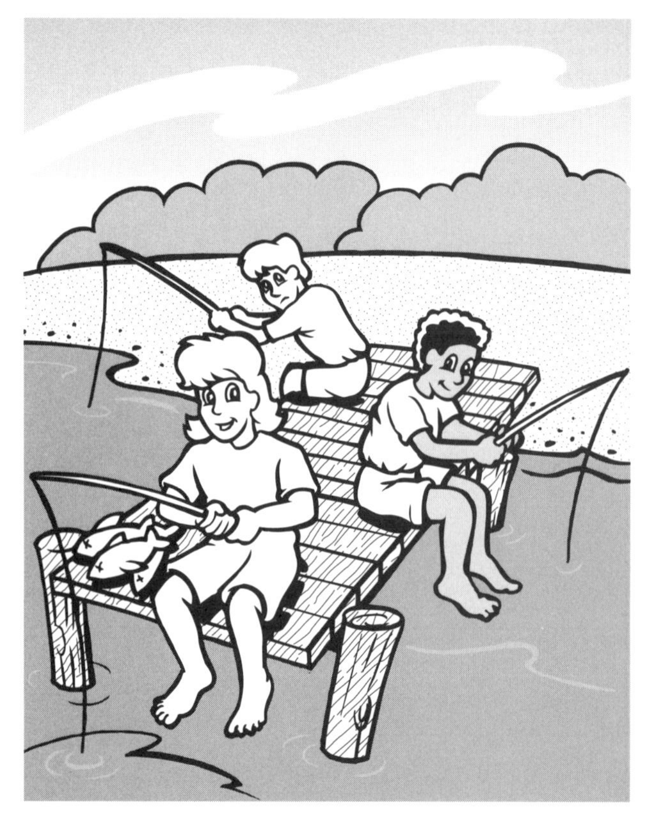

1 2 3 4

- ***Who*** has caught the most fish?
- ***What*** are the children sitting on?

- ***Where*** are the children fishing?
- ***When*** is the best time of day to fish?

- ***Why*** do people like to go fishing?
- ***How*** do you catch fish?

Flying Kites

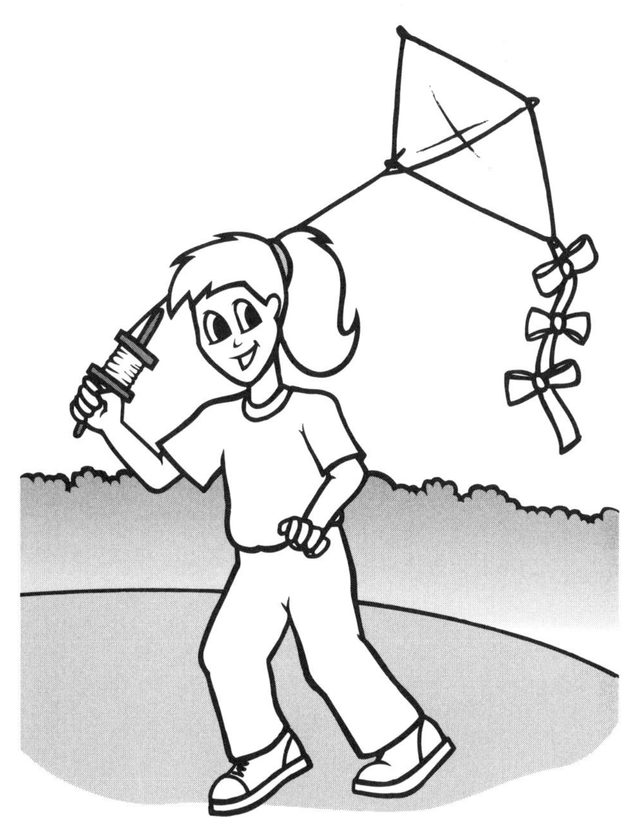

- ***Who*** is flying the kite?
- ***What*** prevents the kite from flying away?
- ***Where*** is the best place to fly a kite?
- ***When*** will the girl stop flying the kite?
- ***Why*** do kites have tails?
- ***How*** does a kite stay up in the air?

1 2 3 4

Frisbees

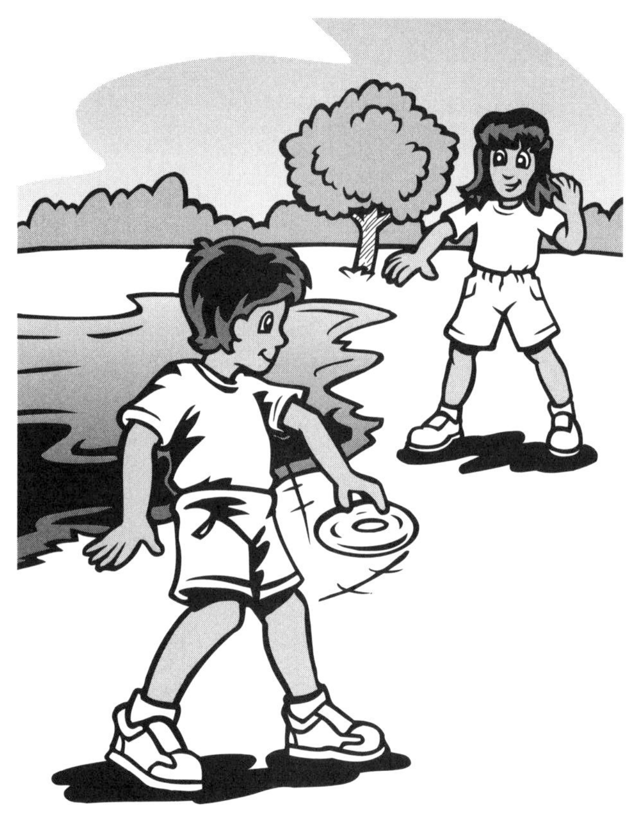

- ***Who*** is throwing the frisbee?
- ***What*** is behind the girl?

- ***Where*** is the frisbee?
- ***When*** do you play outside?

1 2 3 4

- ***Why*** are the children throwing the frisbee outside?
- ***How*** do you catch a frisbee?

Cut on dotted line

Gardening

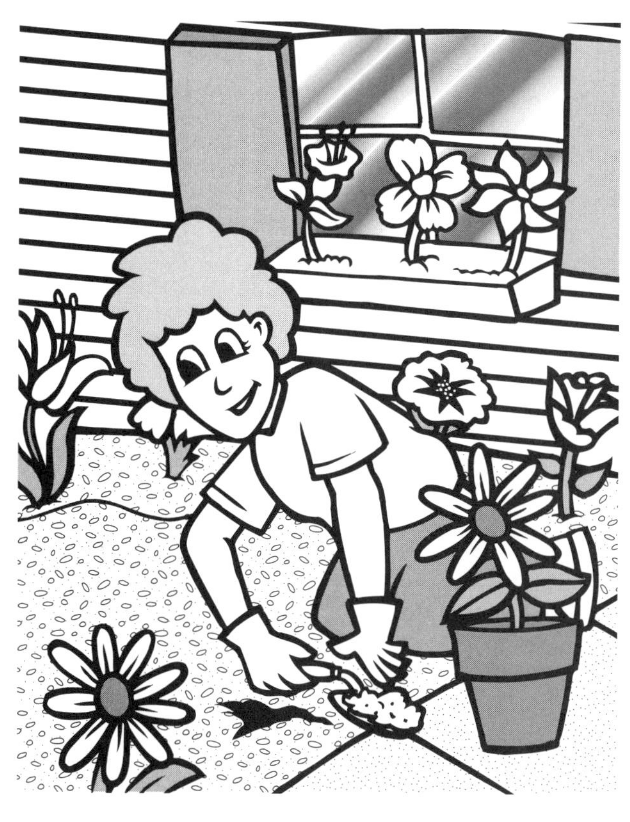

- ***Who*** is taking care of the plants?
- ***What*** is the woman growing?

- ***Where*** is the woman?
- ***When*** is the best time to plant flowers?

- ***Why*** is the woman wearing gloves?
- ***How*** do you grow a pretty garden?

Go-Carts

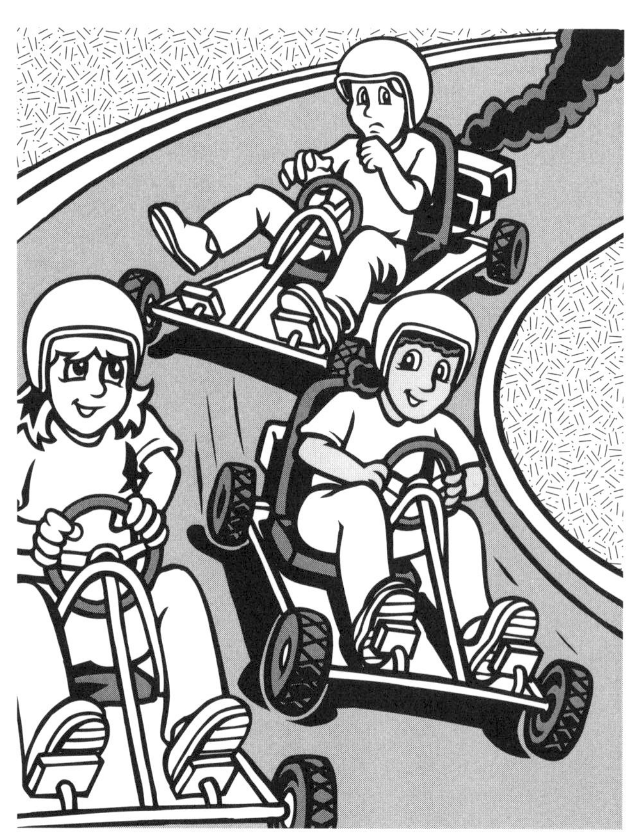

1 2 3 4

- ***Who*** is leading the go-cart race?
- ***What*** are they riding on?

- ***Where*** is the boy?
- ***When*** should the children slow down?

- ***Why*** is the boy in last place?
- ***How*** do you pass another go-cart?

Cut on dotted line

Guitar

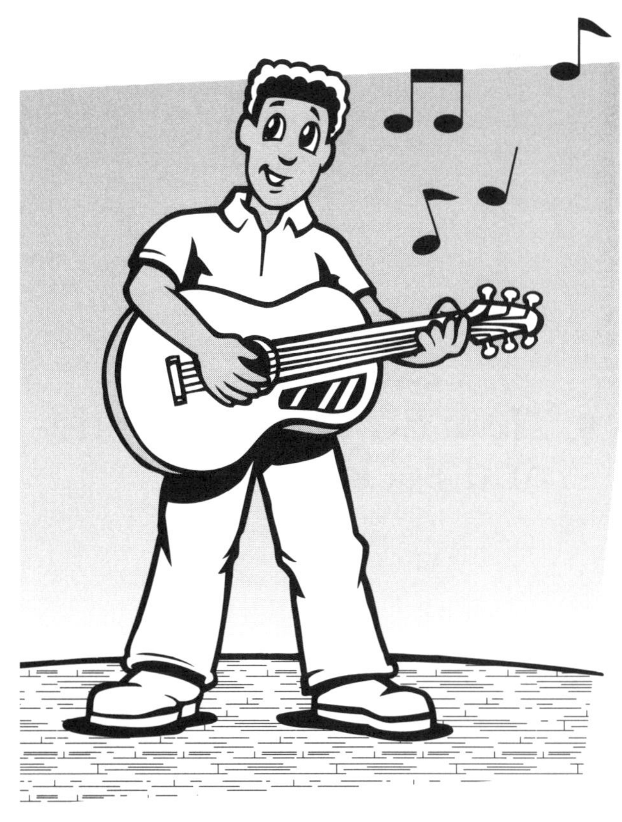

- ***Who*** is playing the instrument?
- ***What*** is the name of this musical instrument?
- ***When*** does he practice?
- ***Where*** is the boy playing?
- ***Why*** does the guitar have strings?
- ***How*** many other musical instruments can you name?

Hide & Seek

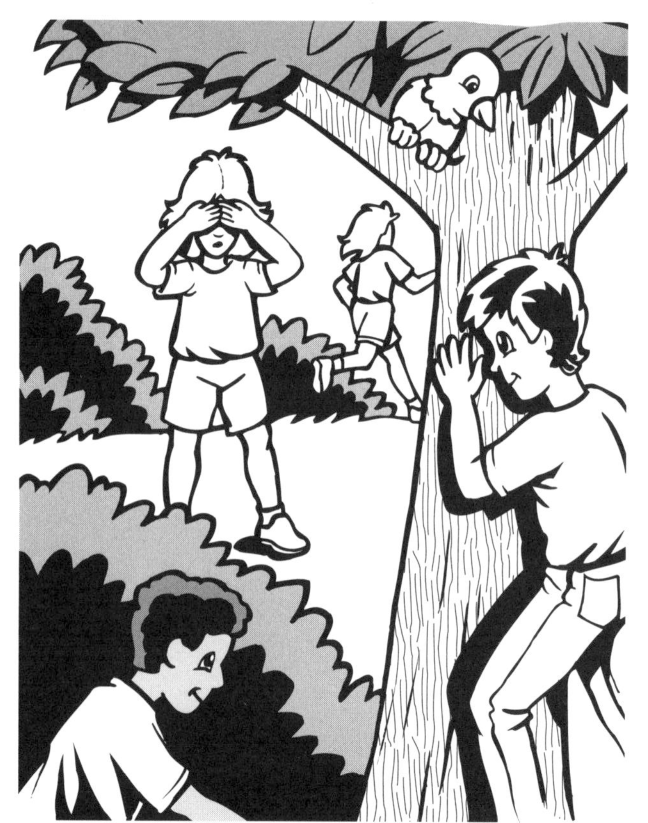

- ***Who*** is counting?
- ***What*** is in the tree?
- ***Where*** is the boy hiding?
- ***When*** will the girl look for the other children?
- ***Why*** is she covering her eyes?
- ***How*** do you play hide and seek?

Hiking

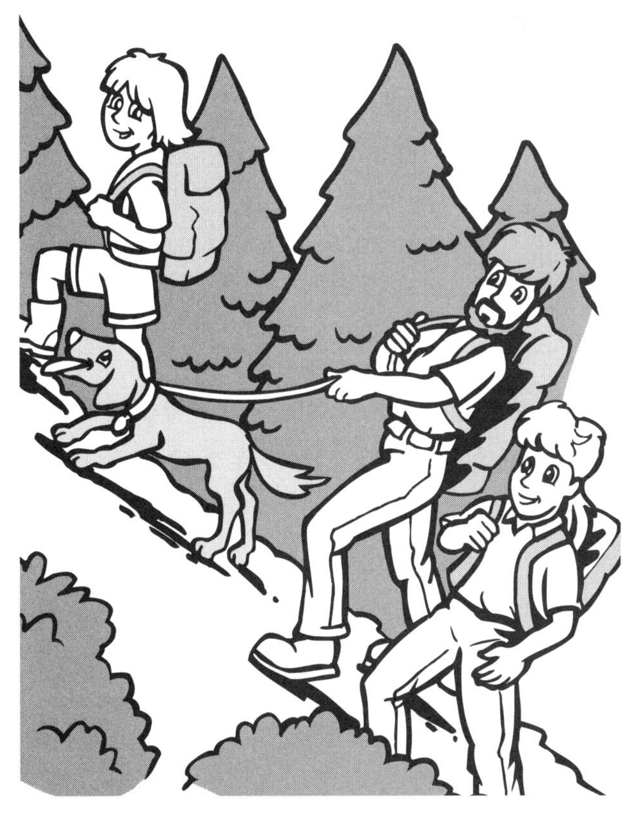

- ***Who*** is in the front of the line?
- ***What*** are the hikers wearing on their backs?

- ***Where*** is the dog?
- ***When*** do people go hiking?

- ***Why*** are they wearing hiking boots?
- ***How*** do they carry water and food on a hike?

Cut on dotted line

Cut on dotted line

Hula Hoop

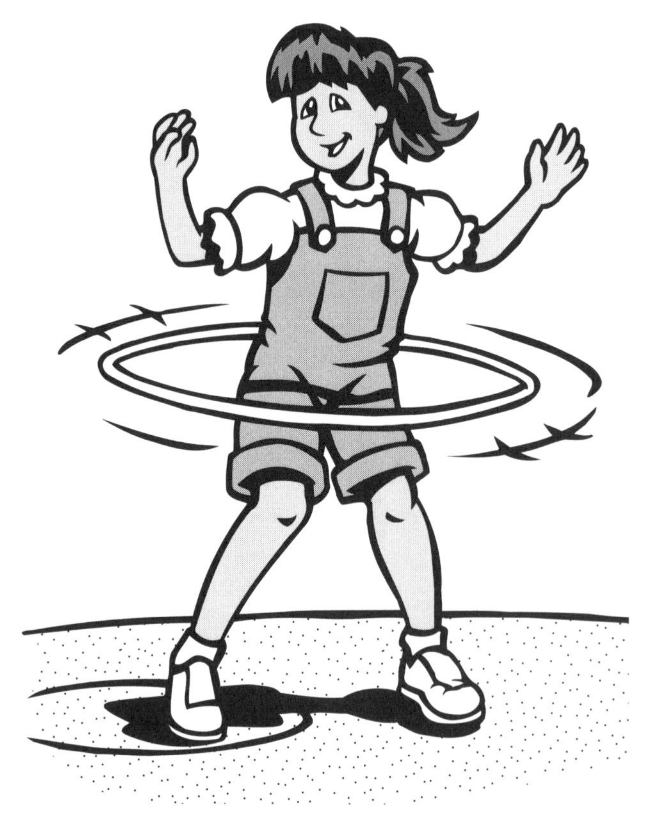

- ***Who*** is playing with the hula hoop?
- ***What*** is the girl wearing?
- ***Where*** is the hula hoop?
- ***When*** will the girl stop playing?
- ***Why*** should she not play with the hoop inside the house?
- ***How*** long could you keep the hoop spinning?

- ***When*** will the girl pick up the stone?

- ***What*** did the girls use to draw the squares?

- ***Where*** are the girls playing?

- ***Who*** is playing hopscotch?

1 2 3 4

- ***Why*** is the girl hopping on one leg?

- ***How*** do you play hopscotch?

Hopscotch

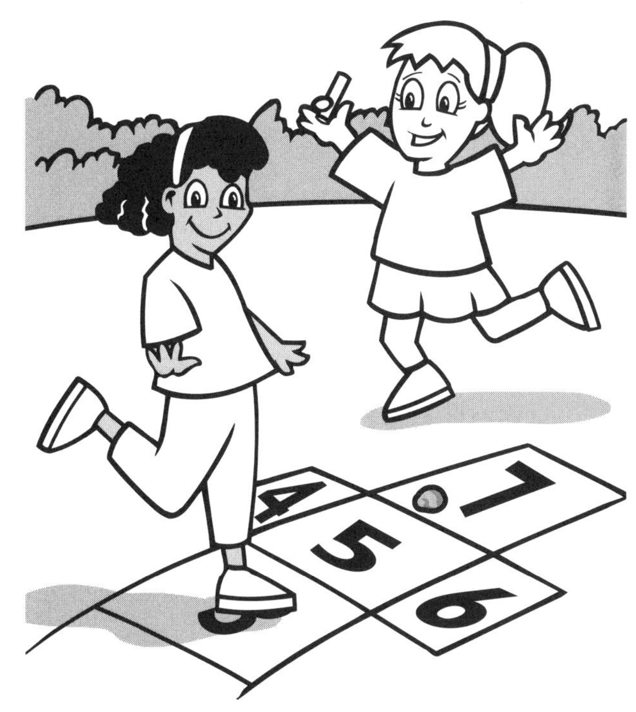

Horseback Riding

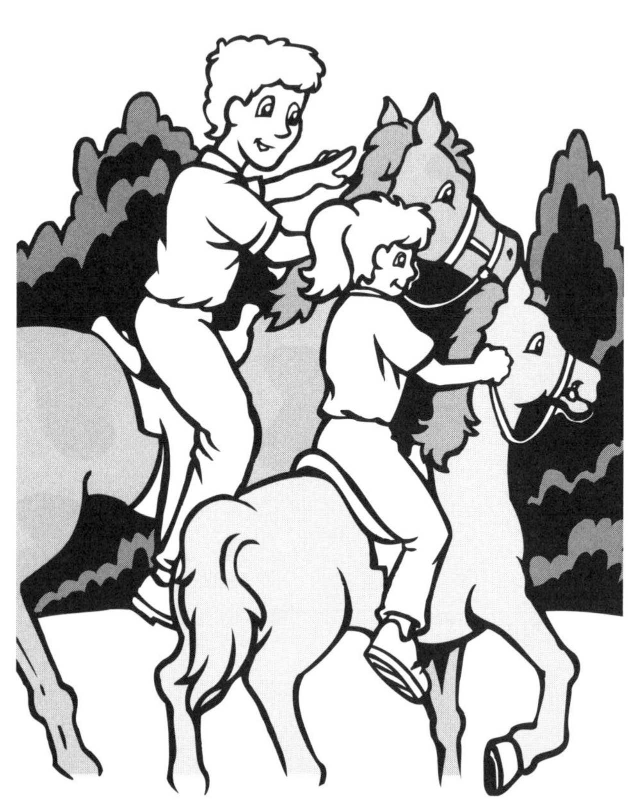

- ***Who*** is on the big horse?
- ***What*** will the people see as they ride?

- ***Where*** are they going?
- ***When*** do the horses eat?

- ***Why*** does the girl have a small horse?
- ***How*** does the horse know when to turn or stop?

Ice Cream Time

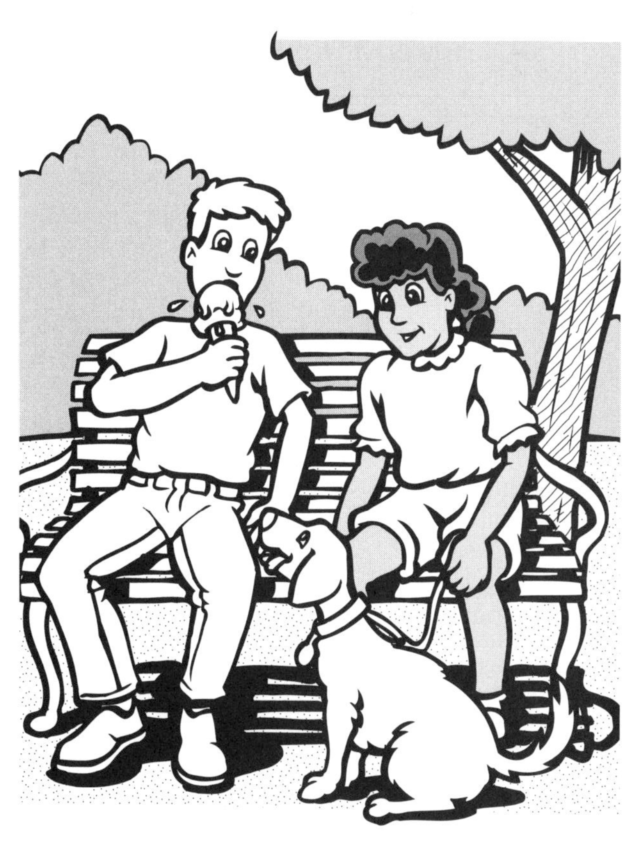

- ***Who*** is eating ice cream?
- ***What*** is the girl holding?

- ***Where*** are they sitting?
- ***When*** do you get to eat ice cream?

- ***Why*** is the dog looking at the boy?
- ***How*** do you eat an ice cream cone?

Ice Skating

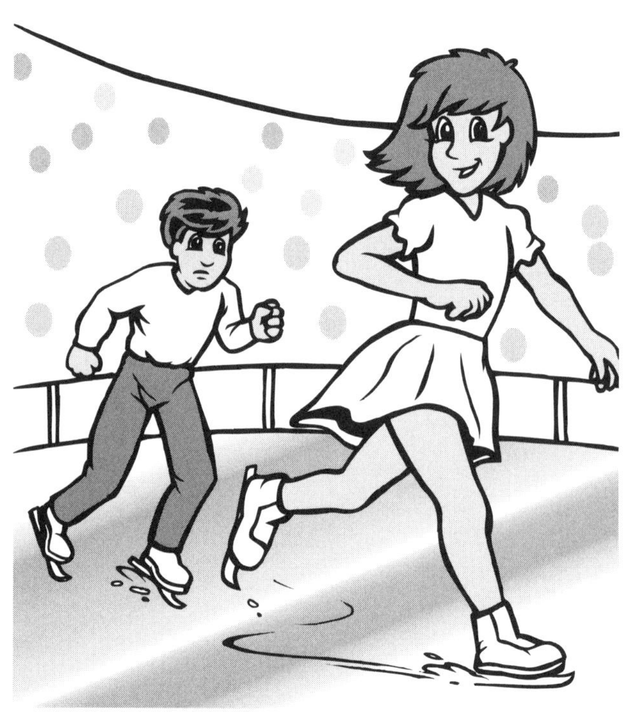

1 2 3 4

- ***Who*** is skating on the ice?
- ***What*** are the children wearing?

- ***Where*** do people go ice skating?
- ***When*** do people go ice skating?

- ***Why*** do people like to ice skate?
- ***How*** do you put on ice skates?

Cut on dotted line

Jumping Rope

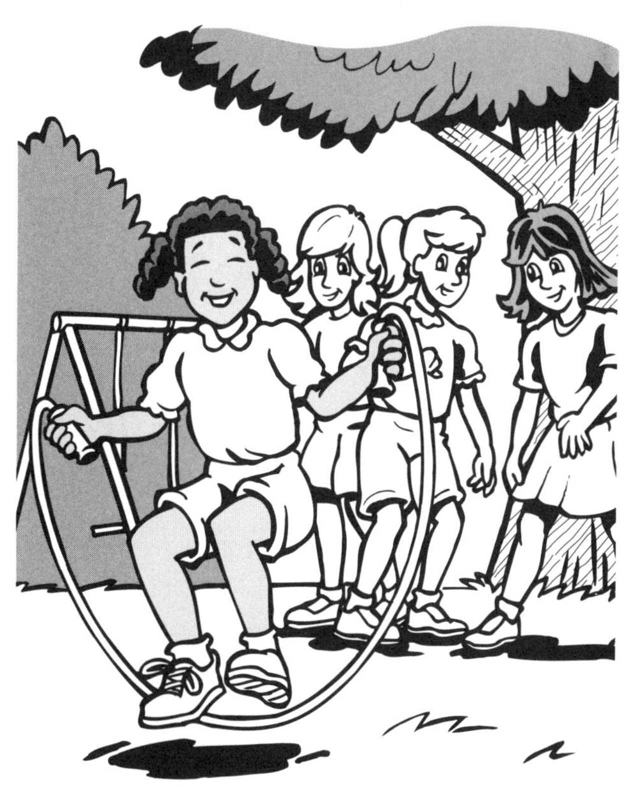

- ***Who*** is jumping with the rope?
- ***What*** is behind the girls?
- ***Where*** are the girls?
- ***When*** will the other children get a turn?
- ***Why*** are the girls taking turns?
- ***How*** do you jump rope?

1 2 3 4

Jumping Over Waves

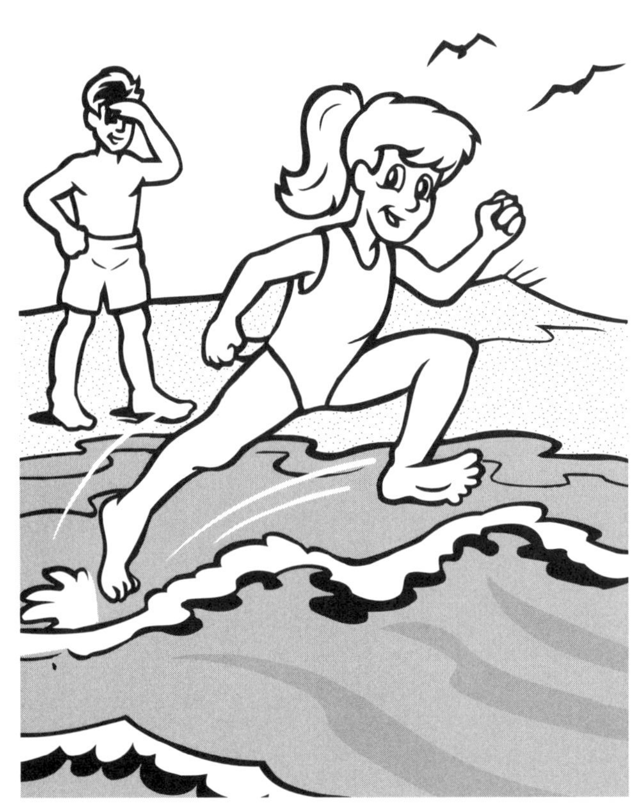

- ***Who*** is on the beach?
- ***What*** is the girl jumping over?

- ***Where*** are the girl and the boy?
- ***When*** do people go to the beach?

- ***Why*** is the boy watching the girl?
- ***How*** do you keep from getting sunburned at the beach?

Cut on dotted line

When do children play kickball?

What is the girl kicking?

Where are the children playing?

Who is watching the game?

3 2
4 1

Kickball

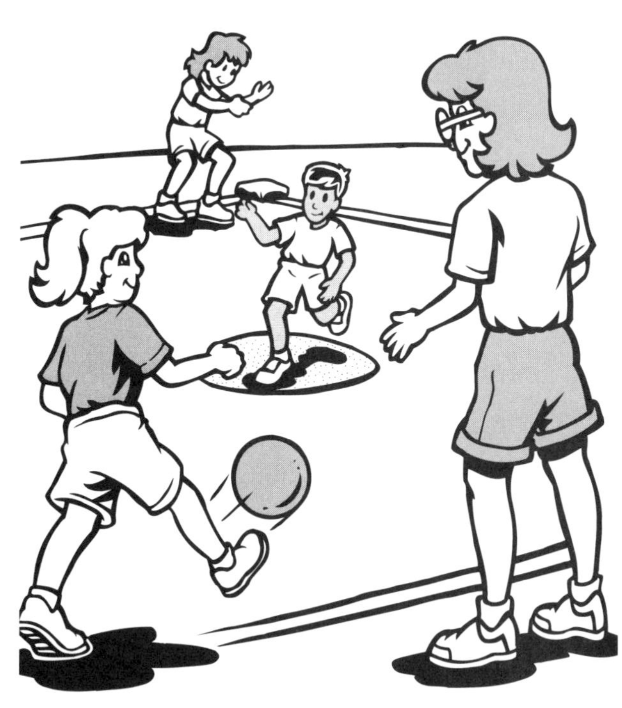

- **Why** do children play games?

- **How** do you play kickball?

Line Dancing

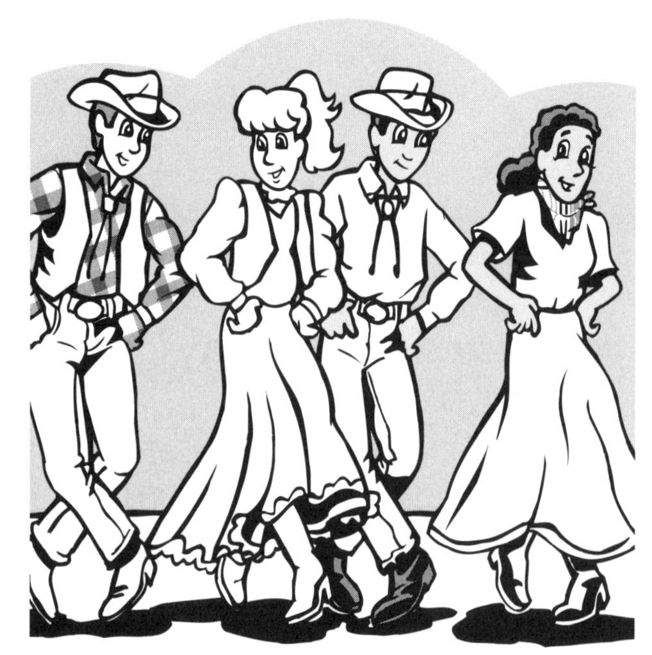

- ***Who*** is dancing?

- ***What*** are the dancers wearing?

- ***Where*** can people learn to dance?

- ***When*** do people like to dance?

- ***Why*** do people dance?

- ***How*** many people can dance in a line?

1 2 3 4

Cut on dotted line

Marbles

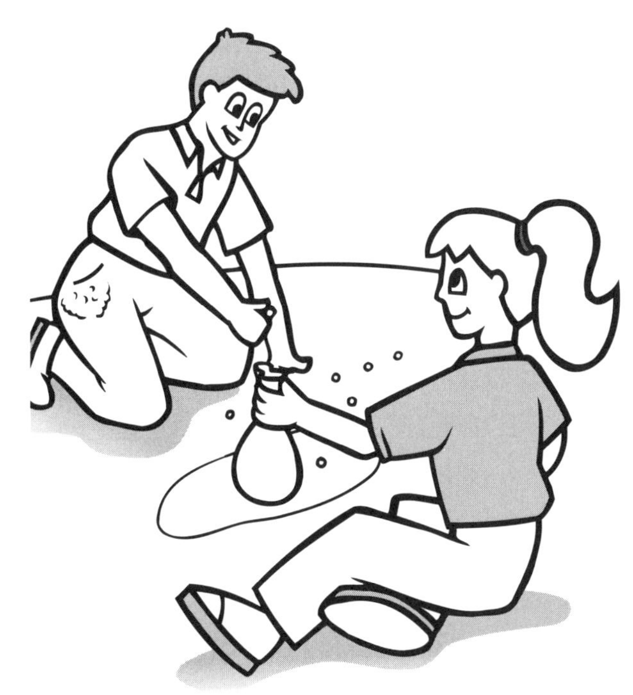

- ***Who*** is playing marbles?
- ***What*** are marbles made of?
- ***Where*** does the girl keep her marbles?
- ***When*** will they finish playing?
- ***Why*** are they playing outside?
- ***How*** many marbles can fit in the boy's pocket?

Cut on dotted line

Model Planes

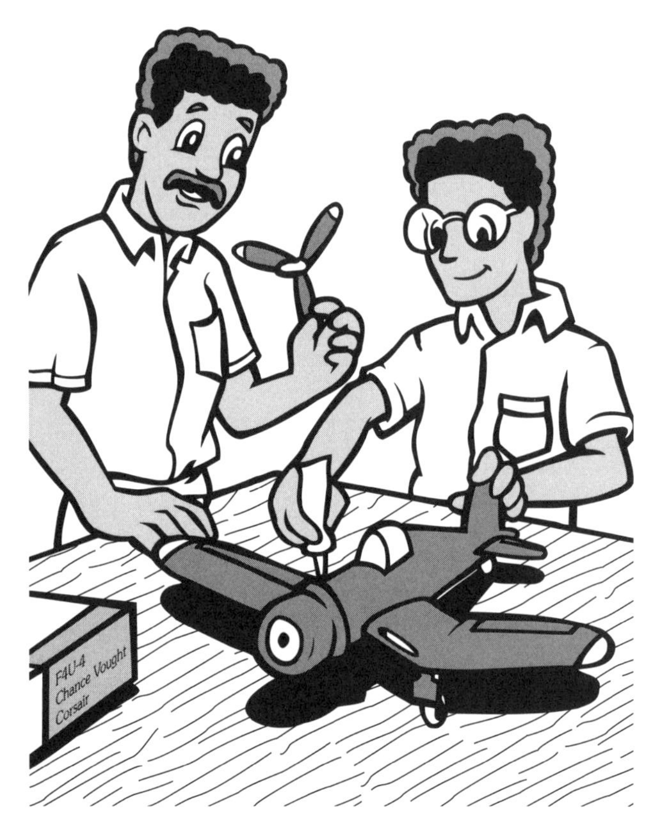

- ***Who*** is helping the boy?
- ***What*** holds the pieces of the plane together?

- ***Where*** do people make model planes?
- ***When*** will the boy be finished?

- ***Why*** is the man helping the boy?
- ***How*** do you make a model plane?

1 2 3 4

Cut on dotted line

Cut on dotted line

- ***Who*** is painting?
- ***What*** is she using to paint?

- ***Where*** is a good place to paint?
- ***When*** will the painting be finished?

2 3

1 4

Painting

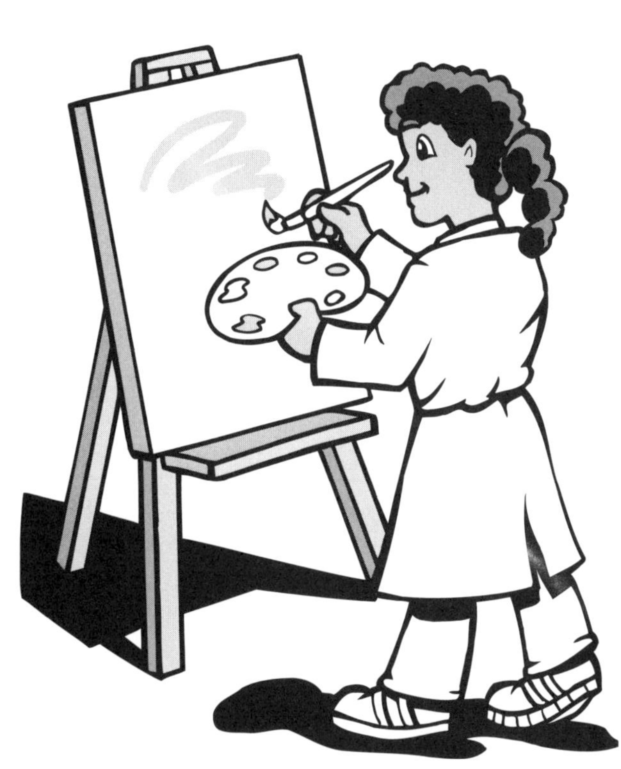

- ***Why*** is the girl wearing a smock?
- ***How*** can she get new ideas for painting different things?

Cut on dotted line

1 2 3 4

Piano

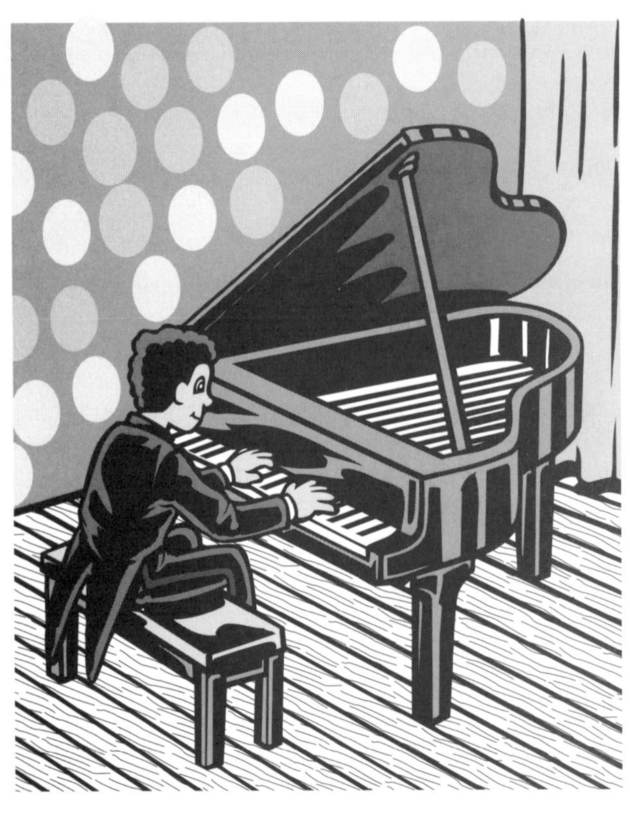

- ***Who*** can play a piano?
- ***What*** is the man wearing?

- ***Where*** is the man playing the piano?
- ***When*** do people practice playing a piano?

- ***Why*** do people go to listen to someone playing a piano?
- ***How*** does a person play a piano?

Cut on dotted line

Playing Catch

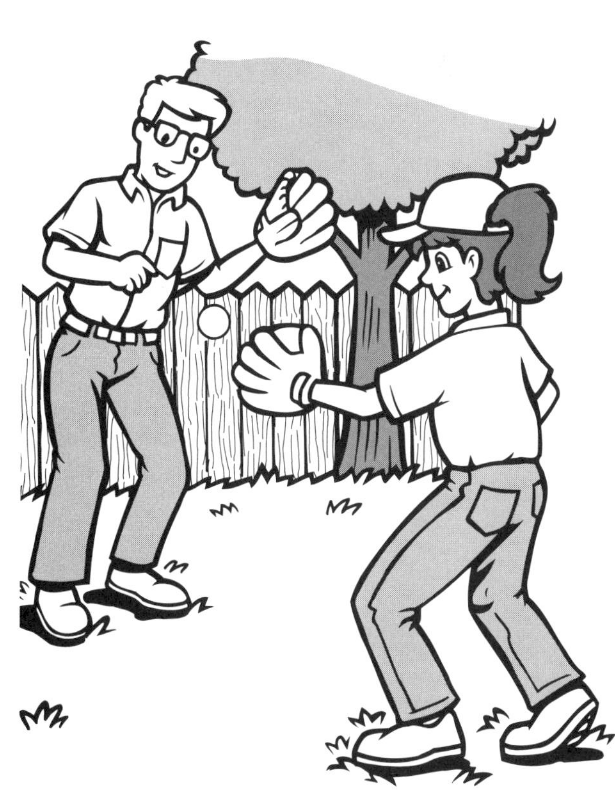

- ***Who*** is playing catch?
- ***What*** are they playing with?

- ***Where*** are they playing?
- ***When*** will they stop?

1 2 3 4

- ***Why*** are they playing catch?

- ***How*** do you know they are having fun?

Cut on dotted line

Pottery

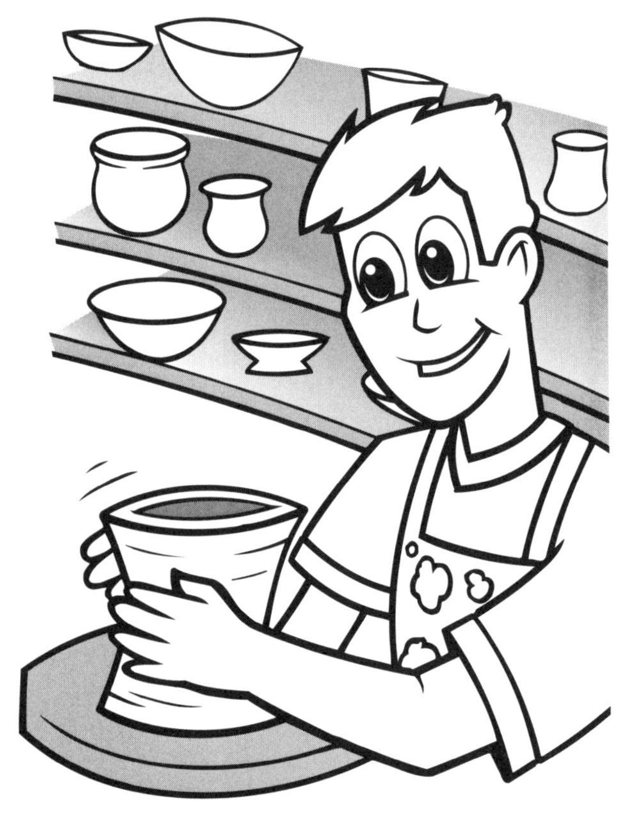

1 2 3 4

- ***Who*** is making the vases?
- ***What*** does the man use to make the vases?

- ***Where*** are the vases drying?
- ***When*** can the vases be painted?

- ***Why*** is the man wearing an apron?
- ***How*** does the clay feel?

Cut on dotted line

Puzzles

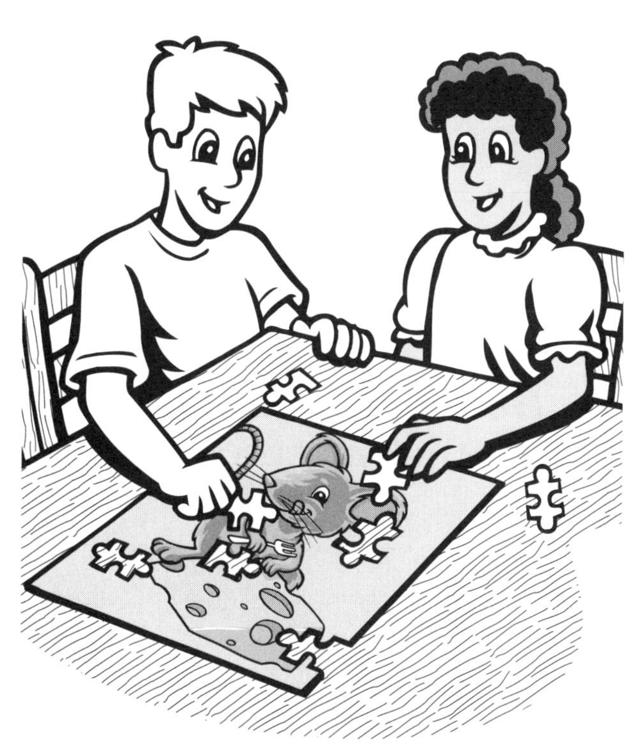

- ***Who*** is putting together the puzzle?
- ***What*** is the best way to put a puzzle together?

- ***Where*** is a good place to put together a puzzle?
- ***When*** will the puzzle be finished?

- ***Why*** do people like puzzles?
- ***How*** many pieces can be in a puzzle?

Reading

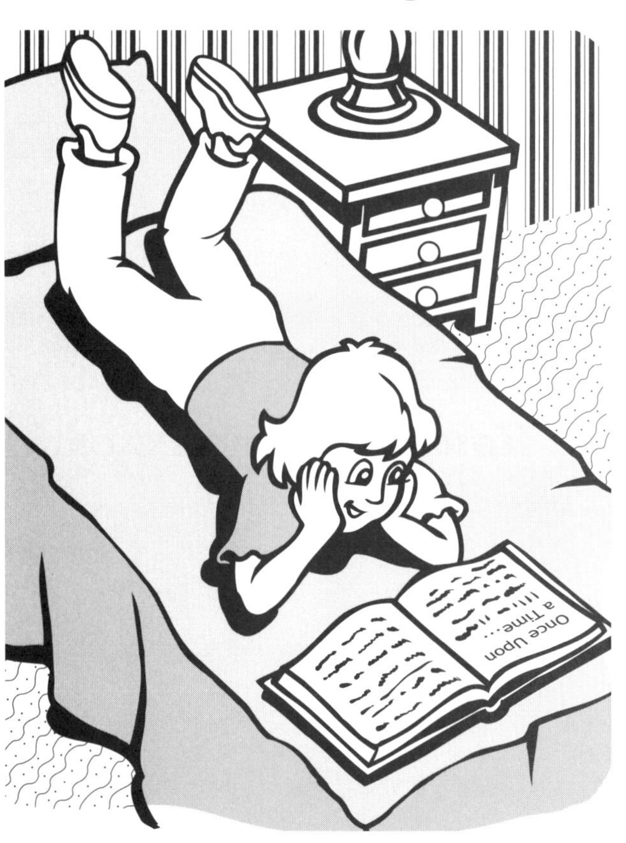

1 2 3 4

- ***Who*** is reading the book?

- ***What*** is the girl lying on?

- ***Where*** is the girl reading?

- ***When*** do you like to read?

- ***Why*** is the girl reading the book?

- ***How*** can you tell she is enjoying the book?

Cut on dotted line

- ***Who*** is climbing the rock?
- ***What*** special equipment is needed to climb rocks?
- ***Where*** is the girl climbing?
- ***When*** is a good time to climb rocks?

Rock Climbing

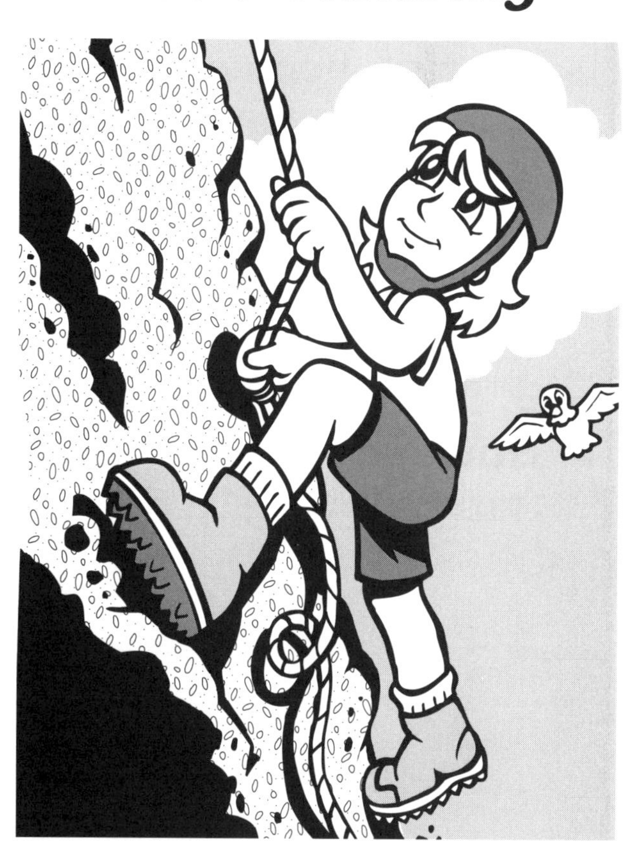

- ***Why*** do rock climbers need special equipment?
- ***How*** difficult do you think it is to rock climb?

1

Rollerblading

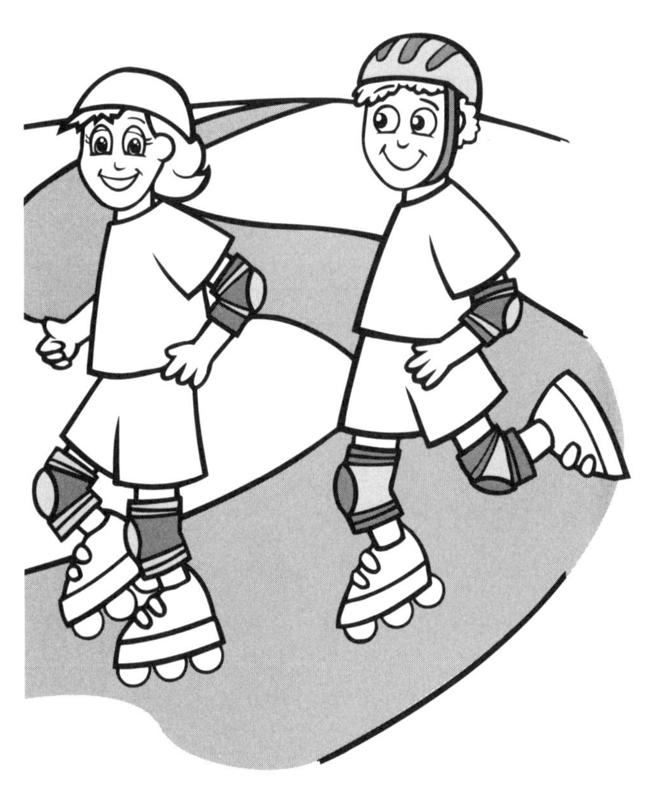

2

- ***Who*** is rollerblading?
- ***What*** are the children wearing?

3

- ***Where*** are they rollerblading?
- ***When*** is a good time to rollerblade?

4

- ***Why*** are the children wearing helmets?
- ***How*** did they learn to rollerblade?

Cut on dotted line

Running a Race

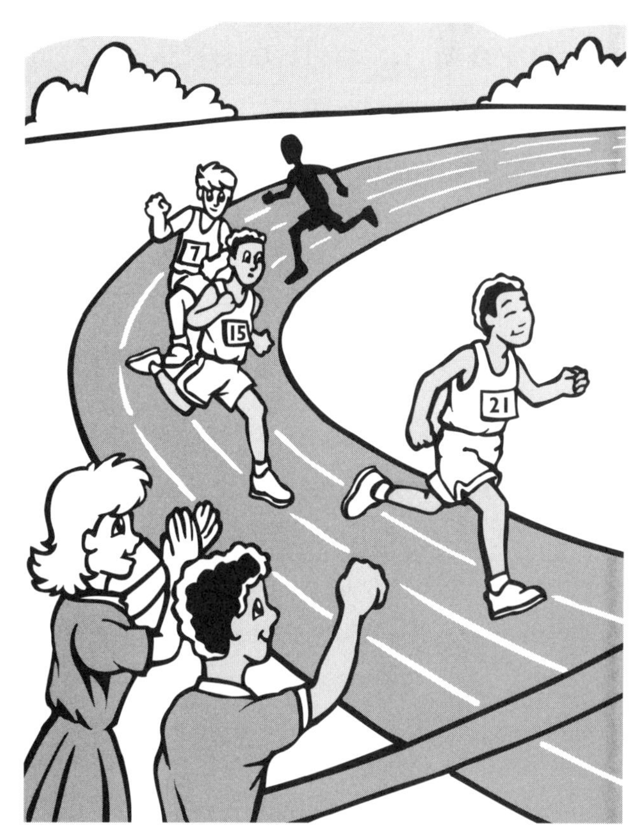

- ***Who*** is in first place?
- ***What*** do the runners have on their feet?
- ***Where*** is the finish line?
- ***When*** will the runners stop running?
- ***Why*** is the girl in the dress clapping?
- ***How*** does a person get ready to run a race?

1 2 3 4

Cut on dotted line

Sailing

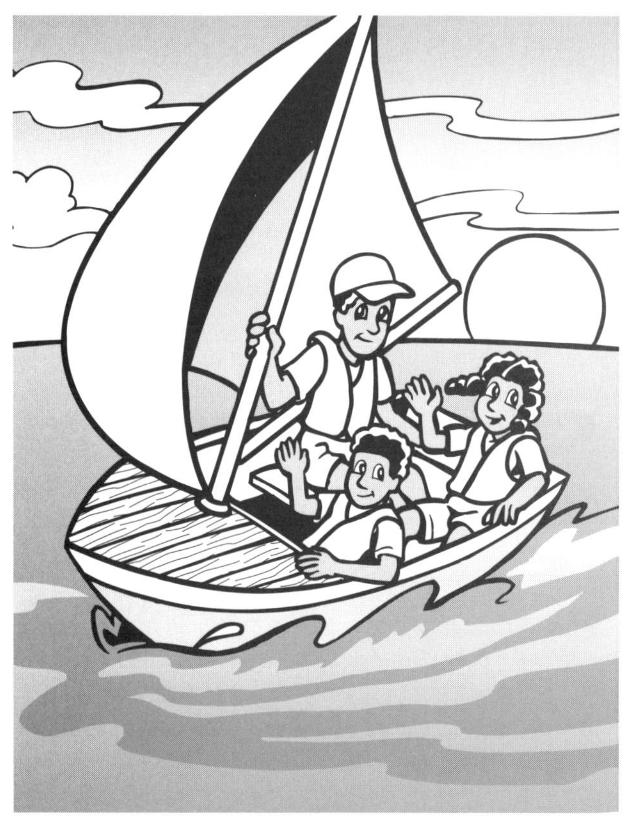

- ***Who*** is wearing a hat?
- ***What*** are the people riding in?
- ***Where*** are they sailing?
- ***When*** will they stop sailing?
- ***Why*** is everyone wearing a life jacket?
- ***How*** does a sailboat move across the water?

1 2 3 4

Sandcastle

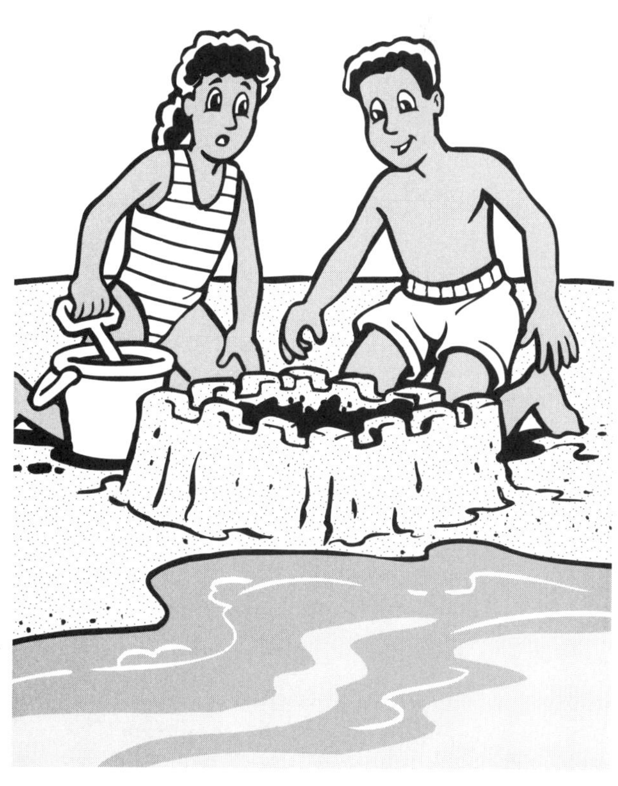

- ***Who*** has the bucket?
- ***What*** are the children making?
- ***Where*** is the shovel?
- ***When*** do children make sandcastles?
- ***Why*** is the girl looking at the water?
- ***How*** do you build a sandcastle?

Cut on dotted line

Skateboarding

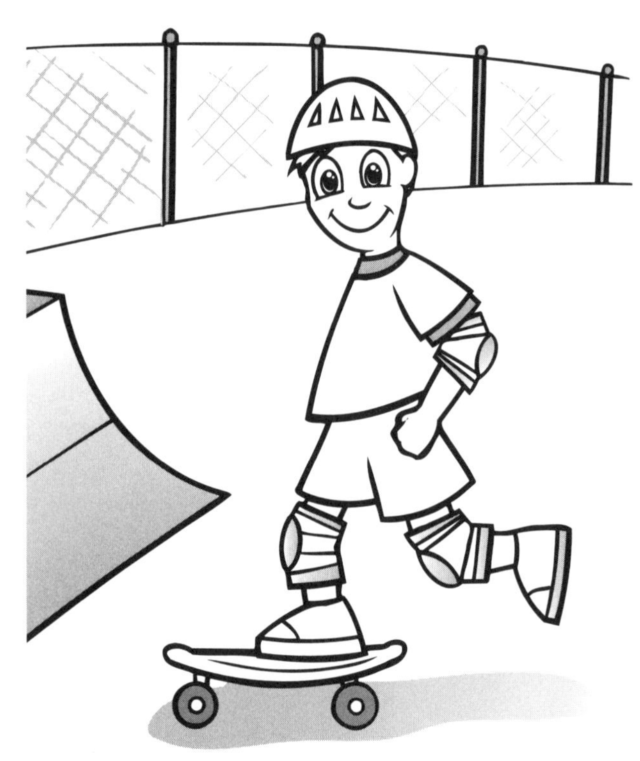

- ***Who*** is skateboarding?
- ***What*** is he wearing?

- ***Where*** is a safe place to skateboard?
- ***When*** will the board need new wheels?

- ***Why*** is it dangerous to ride a skateboard in a parking lot?
- ***How*** does a person learn to skateboard?

1 2 3 4

Cut on dotted line

Sliding

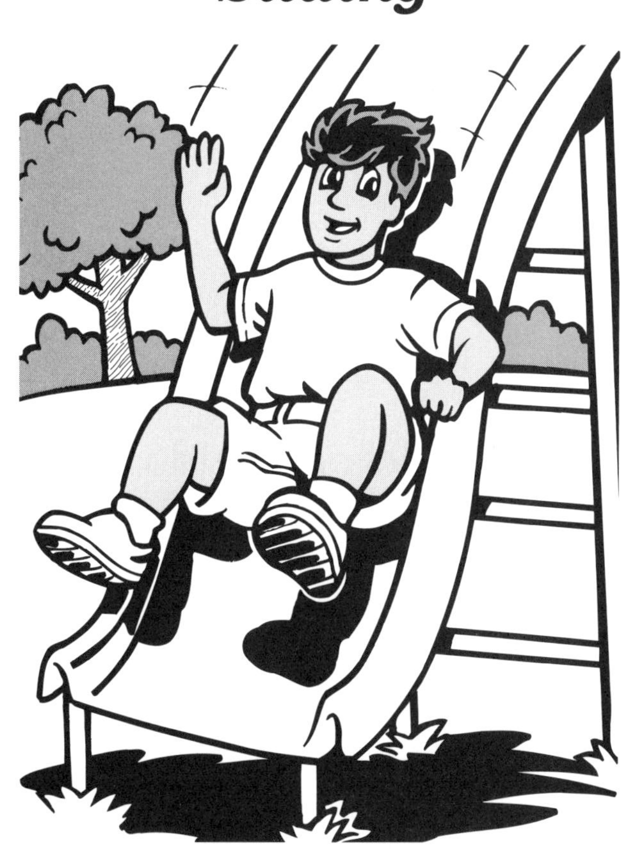

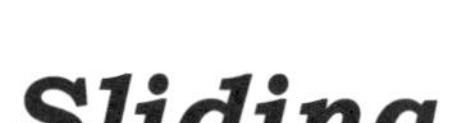

- ***Who*** is sliding?
- ***What*** do you climb to get to the top of the slide?

- ***Where*** do you find a slide?
- ***When*** do people go to a park?

- ***Why*** is a slide tall?
- ***How*** do you climb a ladder?

Cut on dotted line

1 2 3 4

Slumber Party

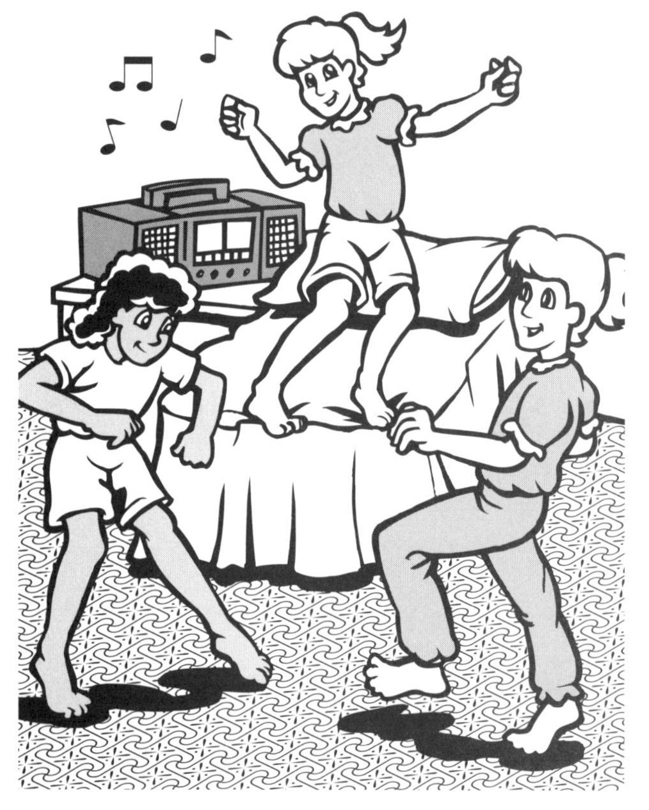

- ***Who*** is dancing?
- ***What*** are the girls listening to?
- ***Where*** are they?
- ***When*** do children have a slumber party?
- ***Why*** are they dancing?
- ***How*** do people dance?

Snorkeling

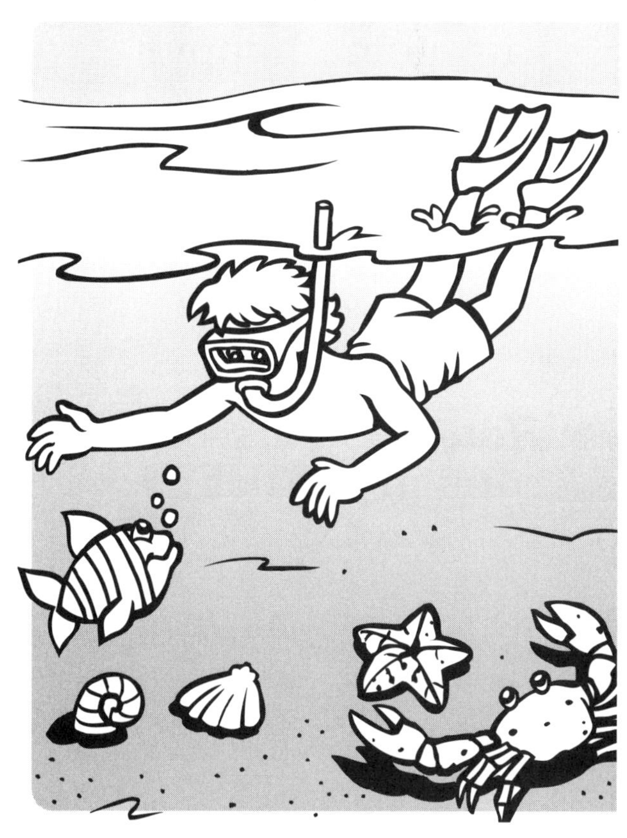

- ***Who*** is snorkeling?
- ***What*** does he see under the water?
- ***Where*** is the starfish?
- ***When*** will the fish swim away?
- ***Why*** is the boy wearing a mask?
- ***How*** do fish swim?

1 2 3 4

Softball

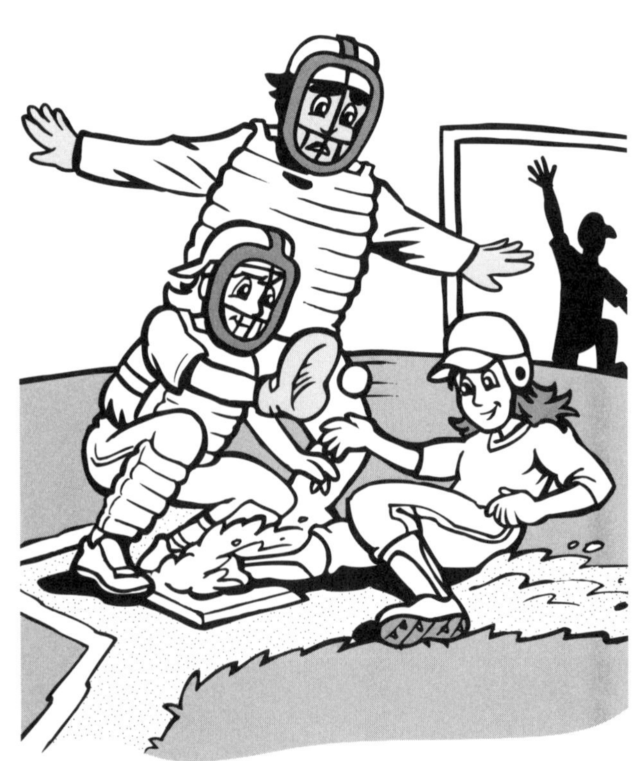

- ***Who*** is playing softball?

- ***What*** is the umpire doing?

- ***Where*** do children play softball?

- ***When*** is a good time to play softball?

1 2 3 4

- ***Why*** is the girl sliding into home happy?

- ***How*** do you score runs in softball?

Cut on dotted line

Stamp Collecting

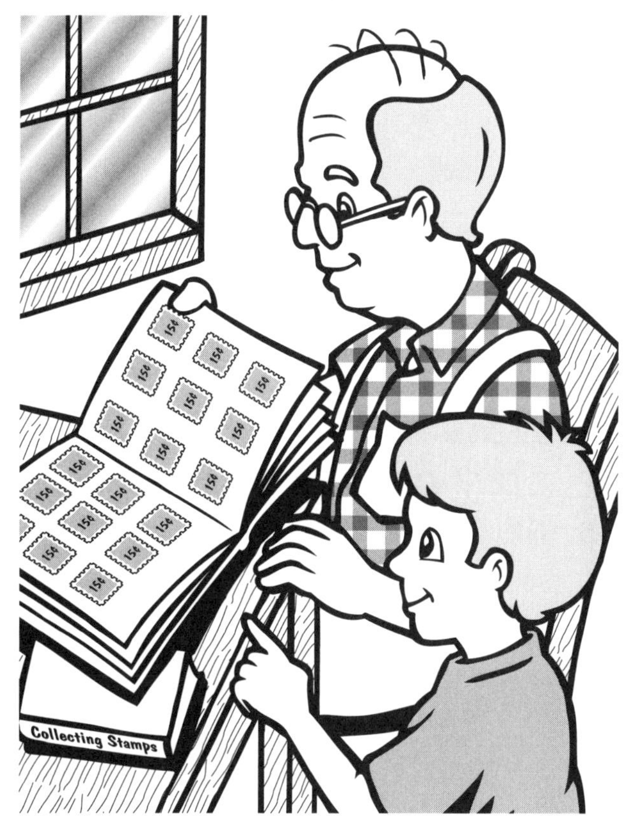

- ***Who*** is looking at the stamp books?
- ***What*** is another use for stamps?

- ***Where*** can stamps be bought?
- ***When*** will the boy put more stamps in his books?

- ***Why*** are stamps kept in a book?
- ***How*** many stamp books can a person have?

1 2 3 4

Surfing

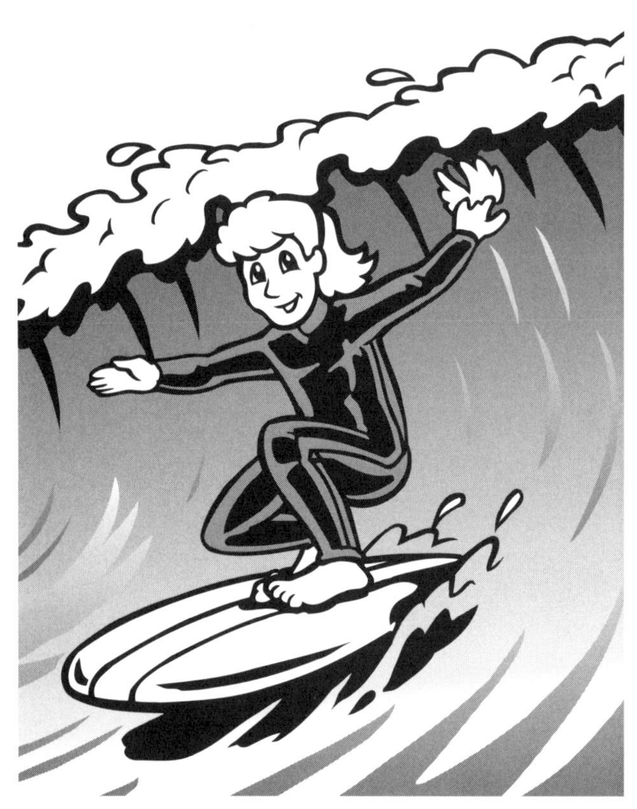

- ***Who*** is surfing?
- ***What*** is she standing on?

- ***Where*** is she riding her surfboard?
- ***When*** do people go surfing?

- ***Why*** is she wearing a wetsuit?

- ***How*** does a person stay on top of a surfboard?

Cut on dotted line

Cut on dotted line

Swimming with a Dolphin

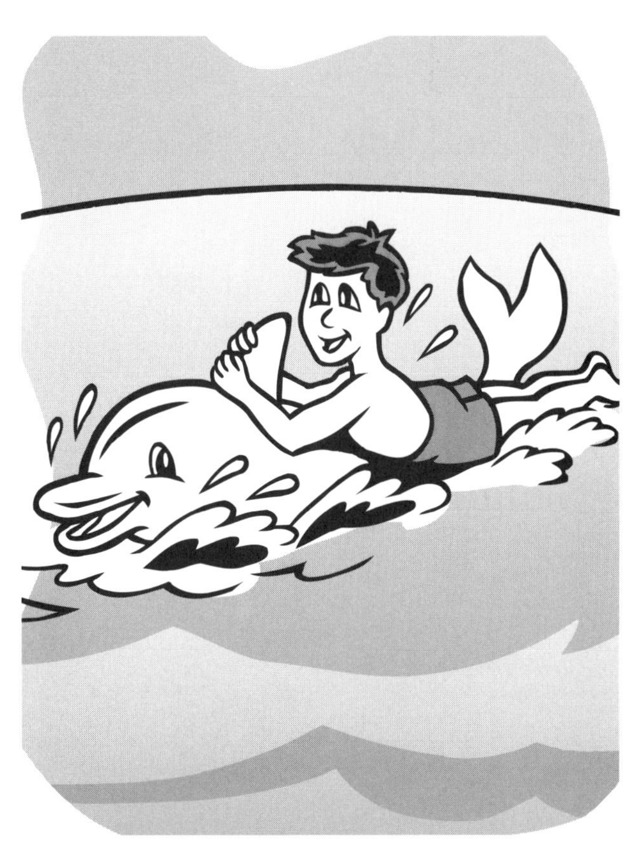

1 2 3 4

- ***Who*** is with the dolphin?
- ***What*** is the boy holding onto?
- ***Where*** are they swimming?
- ***When*** will the dolphin slow down?
- ***Why*** is the boy holding on?
- ***How*** does the boy know the dolphin is friendly?

Swinging

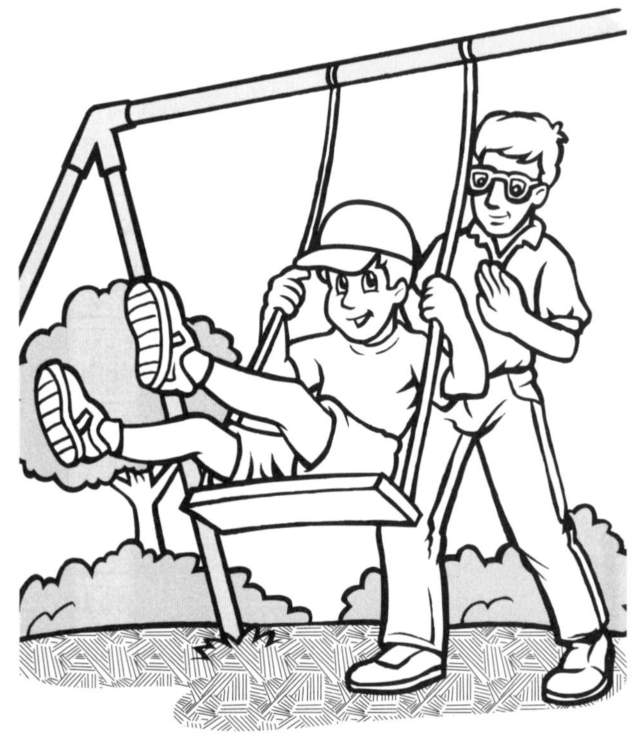

- ***Who*** is swinging?
- ***What*** is on his head?

- ***Where*** is his Dad?
- ***When*** do you go outside to play?

- ***Why*** is he smiling?
- ***How*** does he swing higher?

1 2 3 4

Cut on dotted line

Cut on dotted line

Video Games

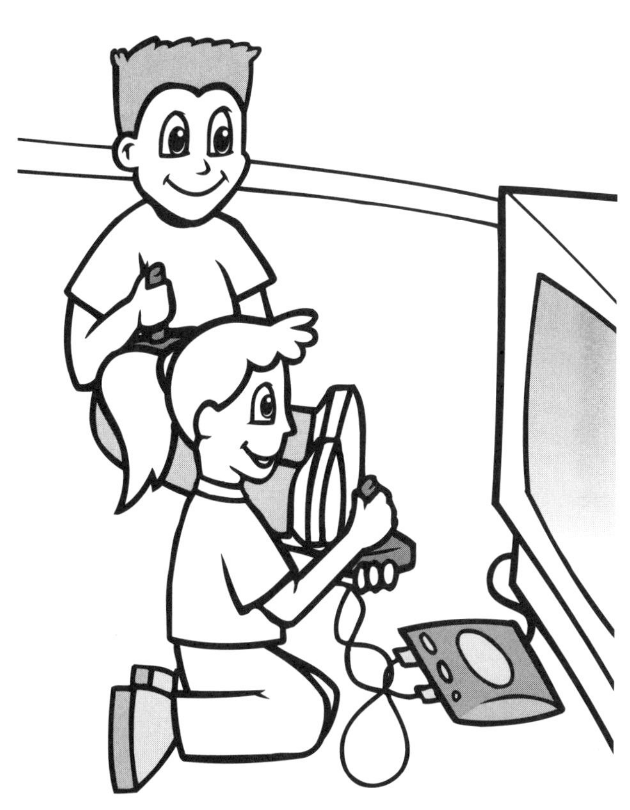

- ***Who*** is playing the video game?
- ***What*** are the children holding?
- ***Where*** are they playing?
- ***When*** is the game over?
- ***Why*** are they playing inside the house?
- ***How*** long have the children been playing?

1 2 3 4

Yo-Yo

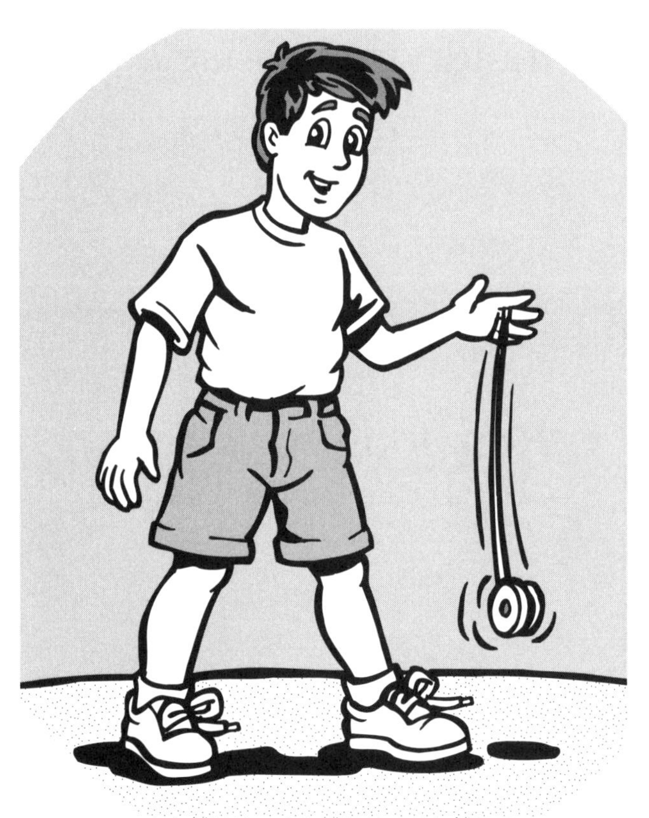

- ***Who*** is playing?
- ***What*** is in the boy's hand?

- ***Where*** can the toy be kept?
- ***When*** does the string need to be wound?

- ***Why*** should this not be played in the kitchen?
- ***How*** is this toy held?

Cut on dotted line

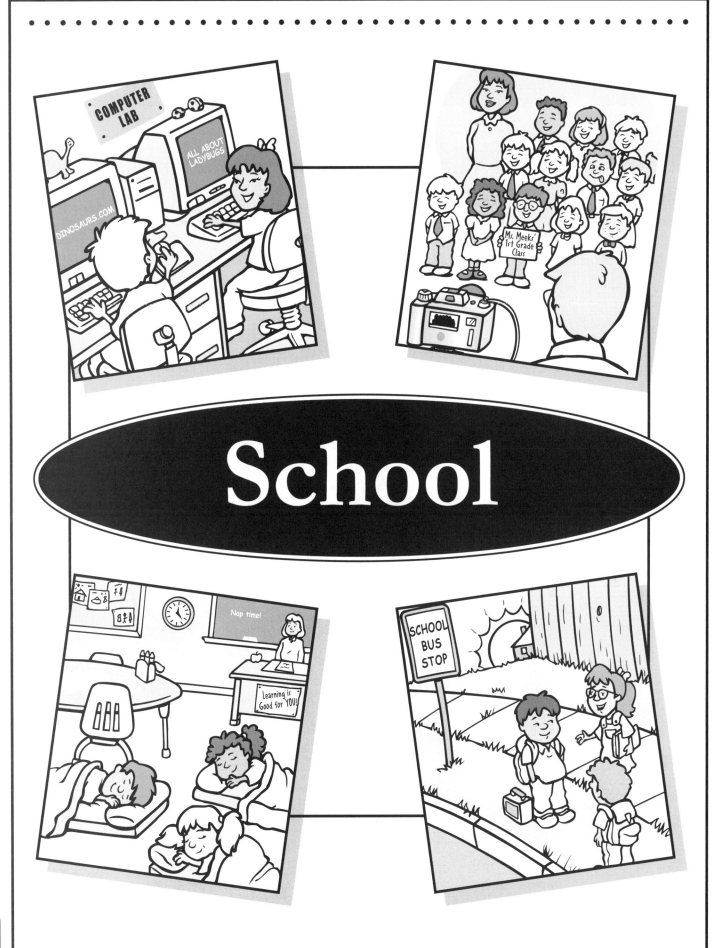
COMPUTER LAB
ALL ABOUT LADYBUGS
DINOSAURS.COM
Ms. Meeks' 1st Grade Class
School
Nap time!
Learning is Good for YOU!
SCHOOL BUS STOP

Circle Time

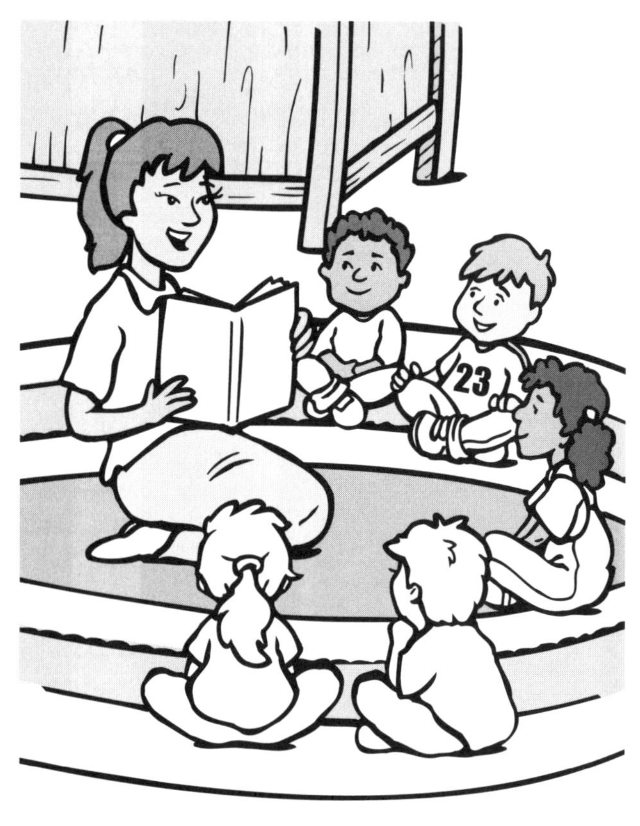

- ***Who*** is reading the book?
- ***What*** is the teacher holding?

- ***Where*** are the children?
- ***When*** is a good time to read a book?

- ***Why*** should the children listen carefully?
- ***How*** are the children acting?

1 2 3 4

Cut on dotted line

Computer Lab

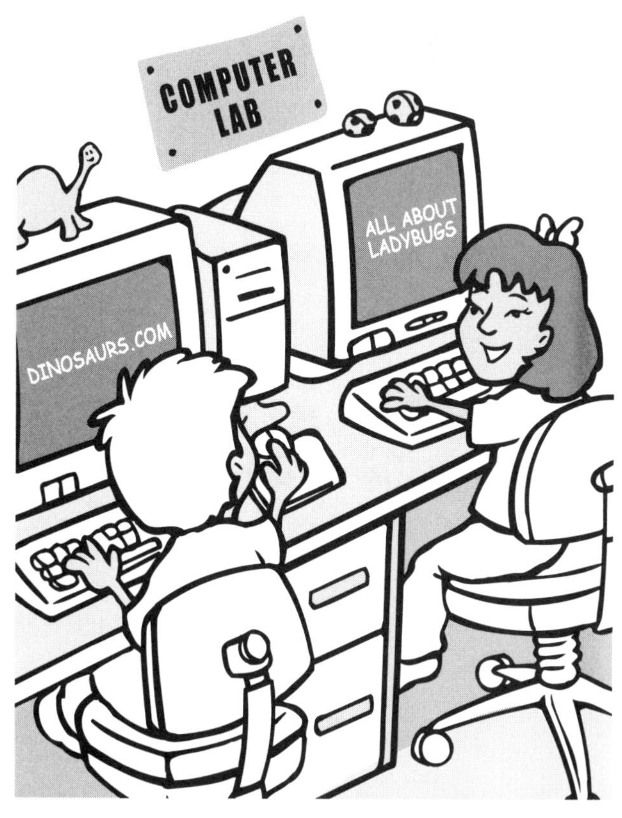

- ***Who*** uses a computer?

- ***What*** are some things to do on a computer?

- ***Where*** are computers found in school?

- ***When*** do students use a computer?

- ***Why*** should children use a computer?

- ***How*** do you turn on a computer?

Daydreaming

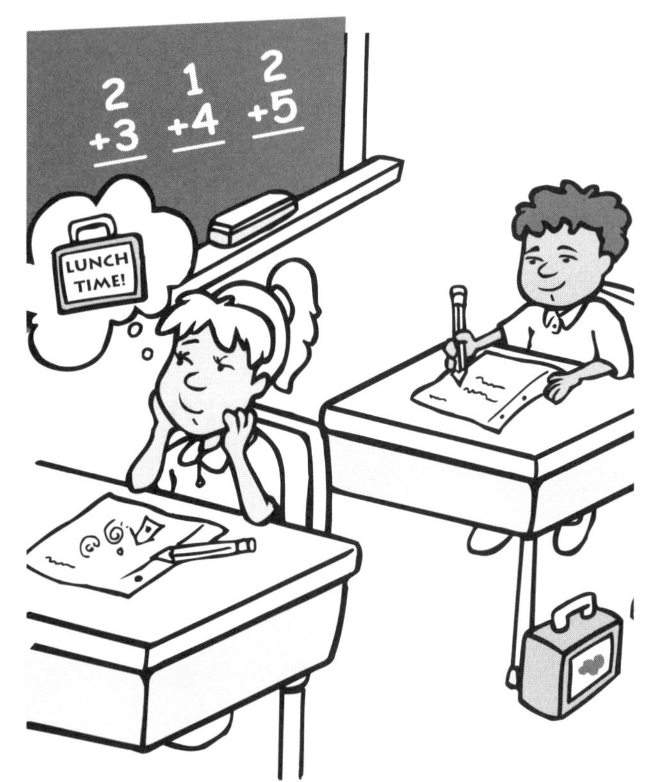

- ***Who*** is doing his/her schoolwork?
- ***What*** subject are the children working on?
- ***Where*** does the teacher write for all to see?
- ***When*** should the children turn in their work?
- ***Why*** is the boy writing on the paper?
- ***How*** do you learn your math facts?

Fire Drill

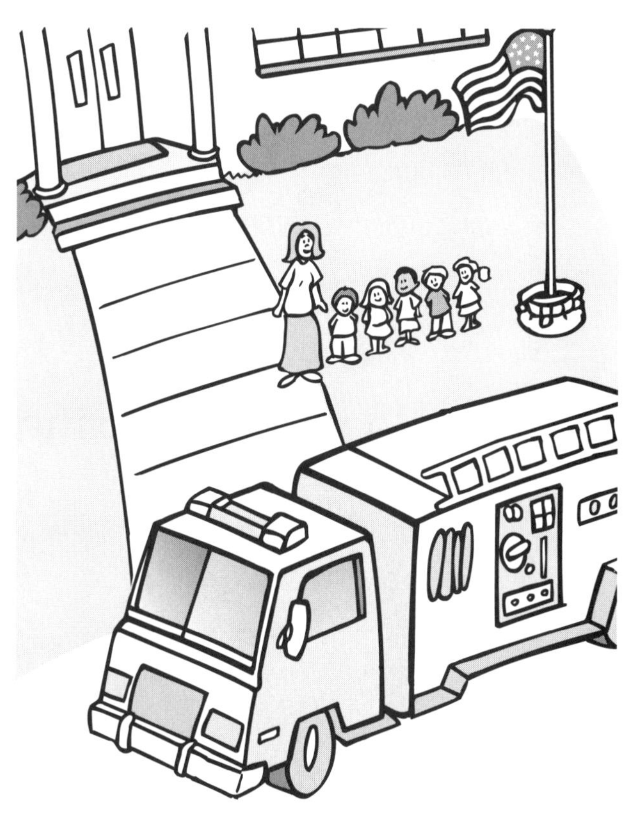

1 2 3 4

- ***Who*** comes to the school when the fire alarm rings?
- ***What*** do children do during a fire drill?

- ***Where*** do the children gather during a fire drill?
- ***When*** do schools have fire drills?

- ***Why*** do schools have fire drills?
- ***How*** do you know it is happening?

Lunch Line

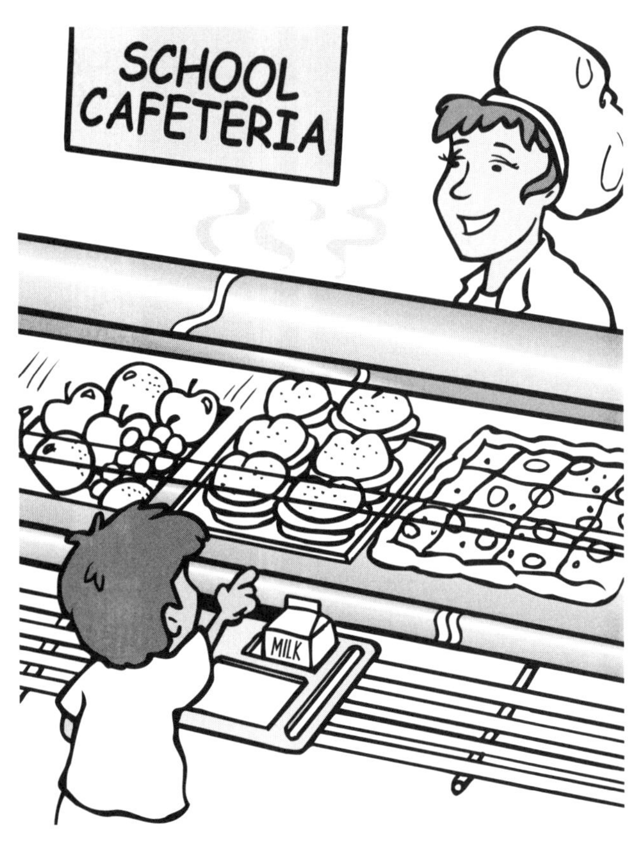

- ***Who*** prepares the food at school?

- ***Where*** do students eat lunch?

- ***What*** types of food are served at lunch?

- ***When*** is lunch served?

- ***Why*** is lunch important?

- ***How*** do you act during lunch?

Music Class

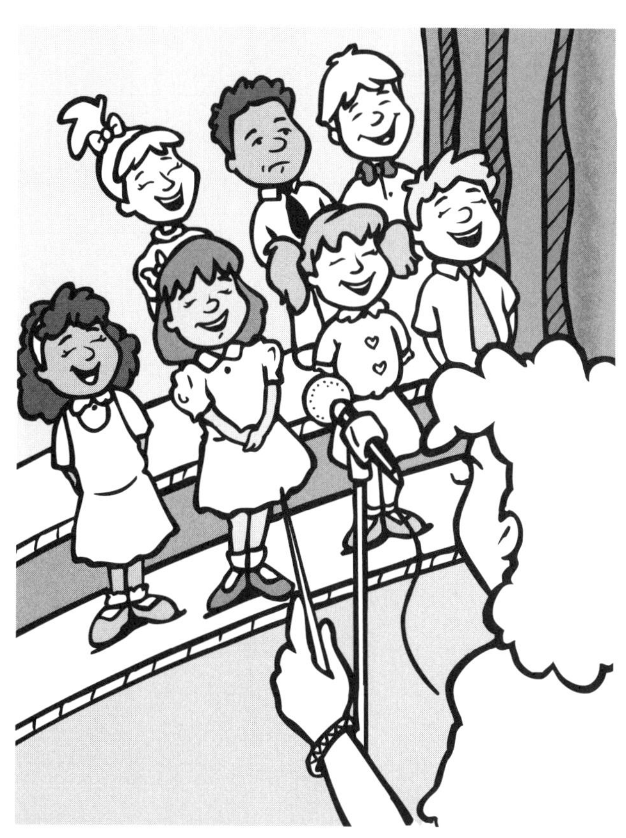

- ***Who*** is in front of the children?
- ***What*** is the teacher holding?

- ***Where*** is the microphone?
- ***When*** is the best time to sing?

- ***Why*** is one boy not very happy?
- ***How*** often do you sing?

1 2 3 4

- ***What*** are the children sleeping on?

- ***When*** is nap time?

- ***Who*** is napping?

- ***Where*** is the teacher?

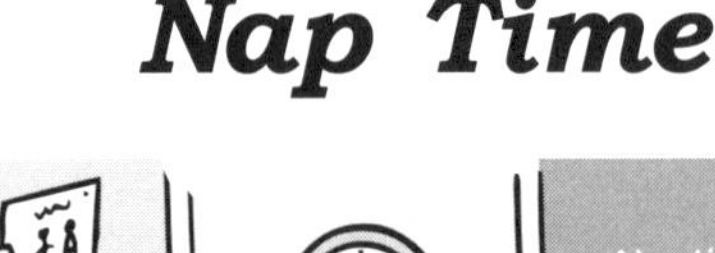

Nap Time

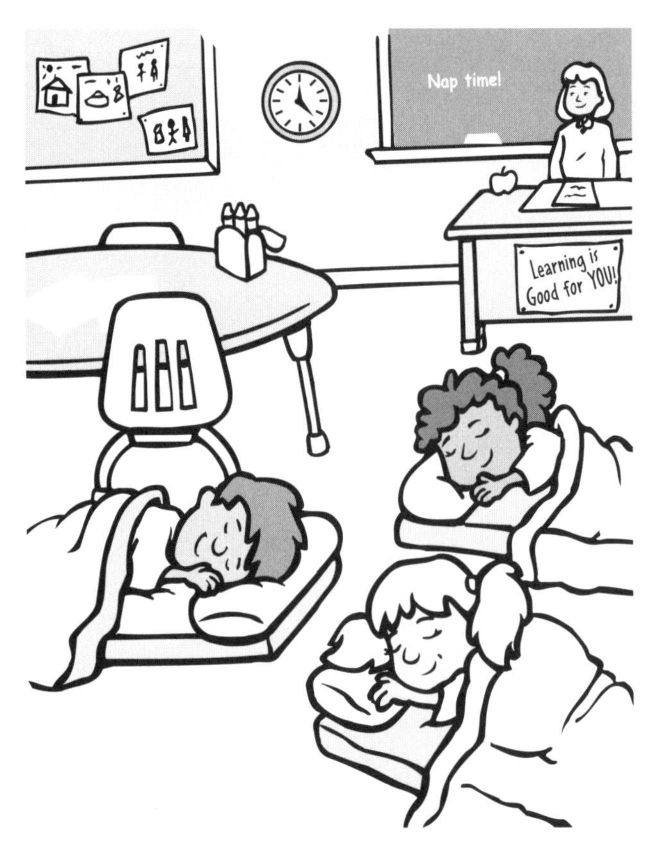

- ***Why*** are they napping?

- ***How*** long will they sleep?

Playground

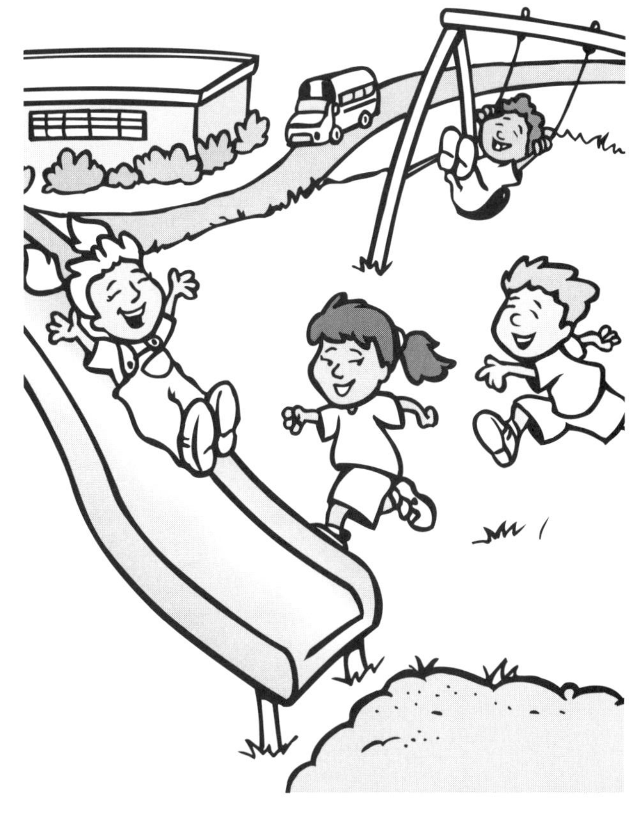

- ***Who*** is playing?
- ***What*** play equipment is at the school?
- ***Where*** do children play at school?
- ***When*** do children play during school?
- ***Why*** do children like playing?
- ***How*** do children know when to return to class?

Cut on dotted line

School

The Principal

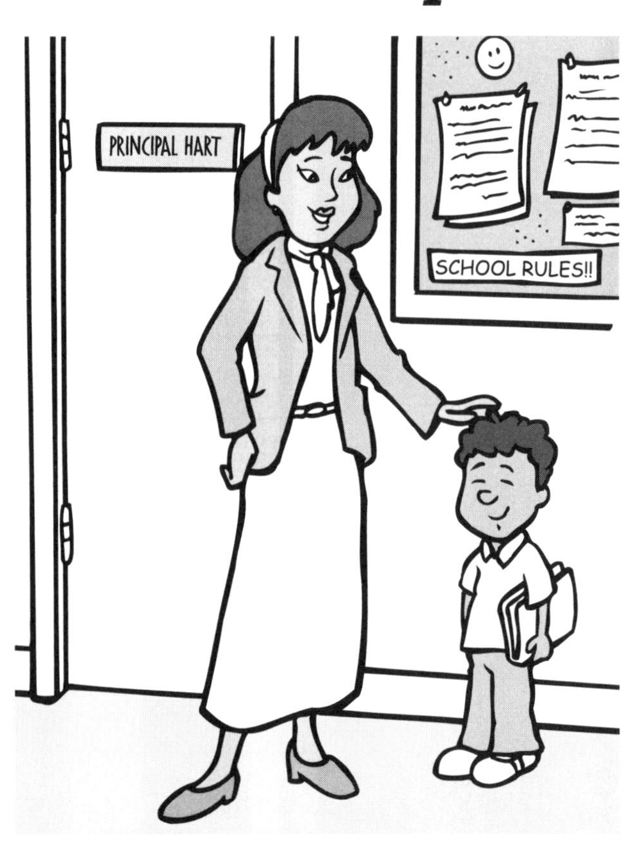

- ***Who*** is in charge of the school?

- ***What*** is the principal saying to the boy?

- ***Where*** is the principal during the school day?

- ***When*** do children see the principal?

- ***Why*** does a school need a principal?

- ***How*** can a principal help children?

School Bus

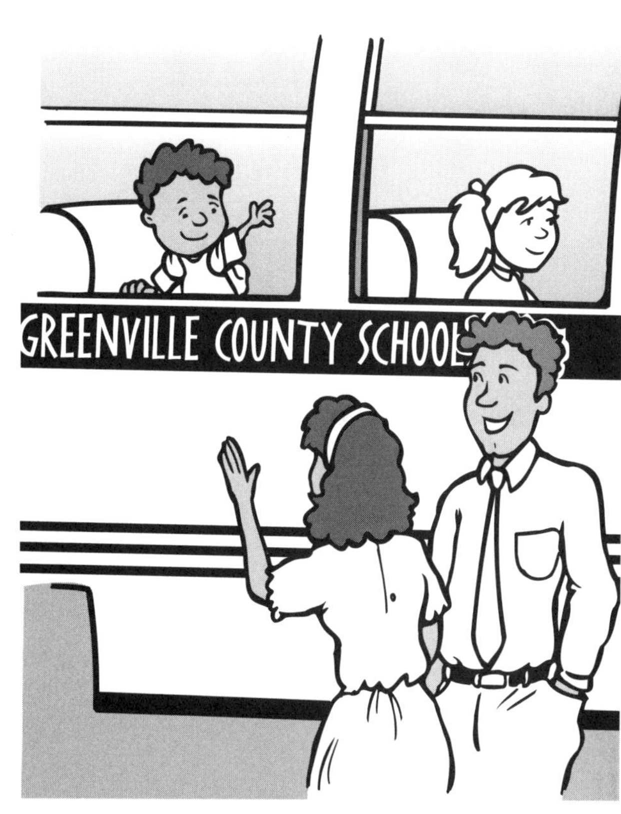

- ***Who*** rides on a school bus?
- ***What*** is the boy doing?

- ***Where*** is the little girl?
- ***When*** will the bus leave?

- ***Why*** are the boy's parents waving?
- ***How*** should his behavior be on the bus?

School Bus Stop

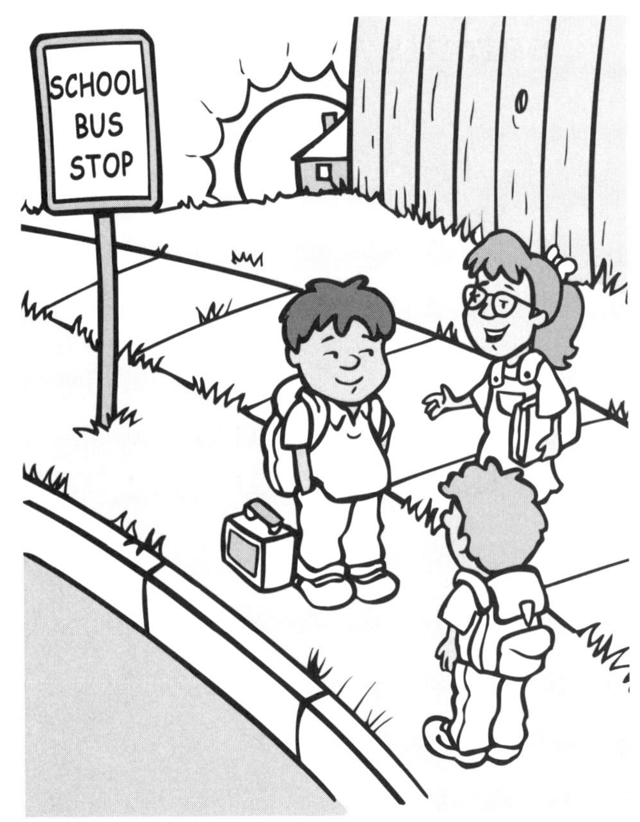

- ***Who*** is waiting at the bus stop?
- ***What*** are they doing while they wait?

- ***Where*** will the bus take the children?
- ***When*** do children wait at the stop?

- ***Why*** do some children walk to school?
- ***How*** do you get to school?

1 2 3 4

Cut on dotted line

School Janitor

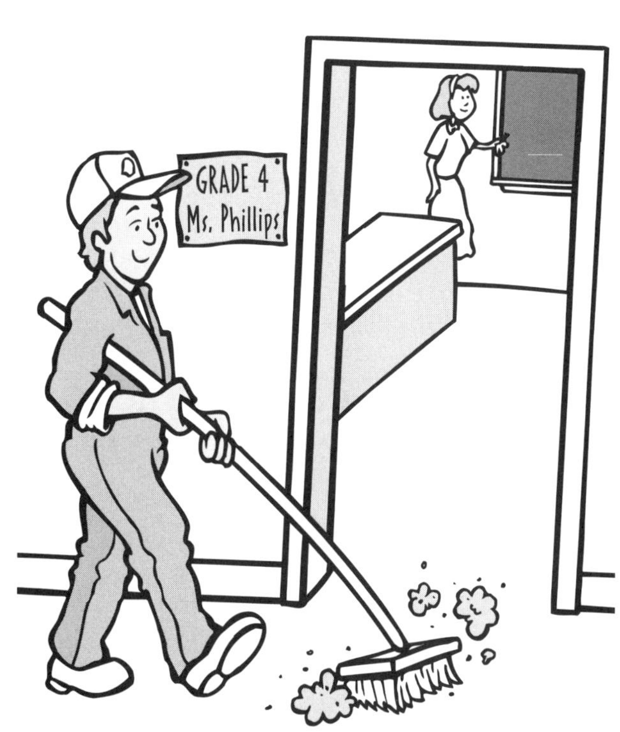

- ***Who*** keeps a school clean?
- ***What*** is the man doing?
- ***Where*** does the man keep his cleaning things?
- ***When*** does the man clean?
- ***Why*** is this man's job important?
- ***How*** can students help this man?

School Library

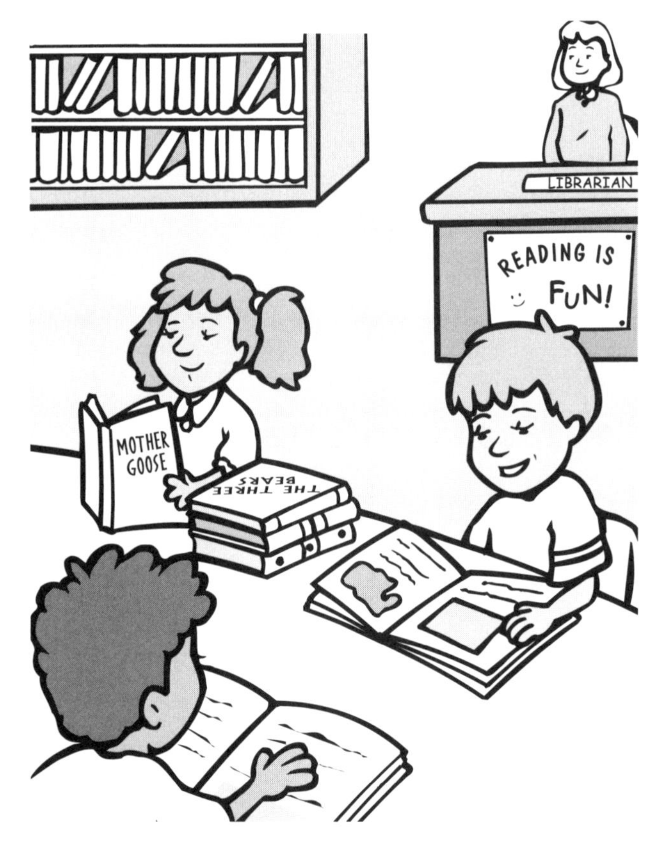

- ***Who*** is in charge of the library?
- ***What*** are some other things besides books found at the library?

- ***Where*** are books kept in the library?
- ***When*** do students use the library?

- ***Why*** should children be quiet in the library?
- ***How*** do children locate a book in the library?

1 2 3 4

Cut on dotted line

Cut on dotted line

1 4
2 3

School Nurse

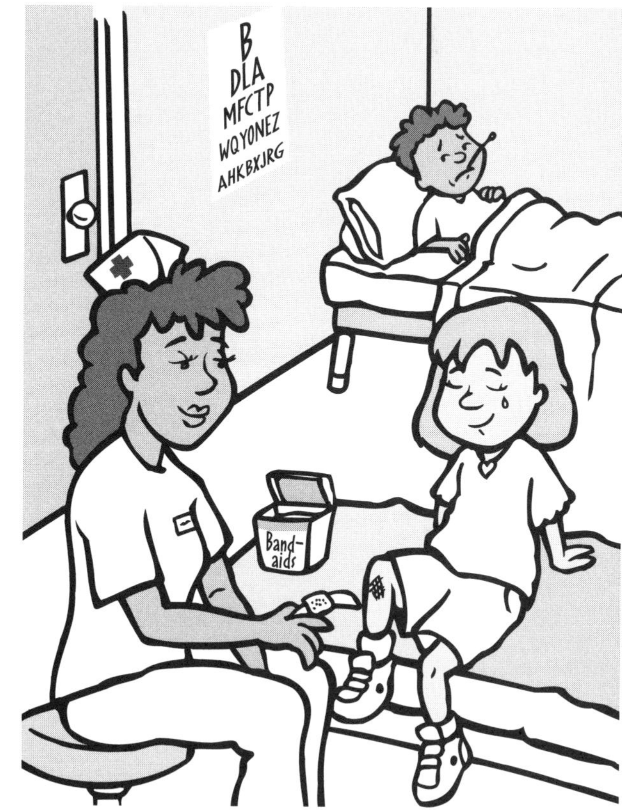

- ***Who*** takes care of sick children at school?
- ***What*** is in the sick child's mouth?

- ***Where*** did the child injure herself?
- ***When*** do children go to the health room?

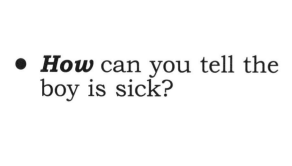

- ***Why*** does a school have a health room?
- ***How*** can you tell the boy is sick?

School Picture

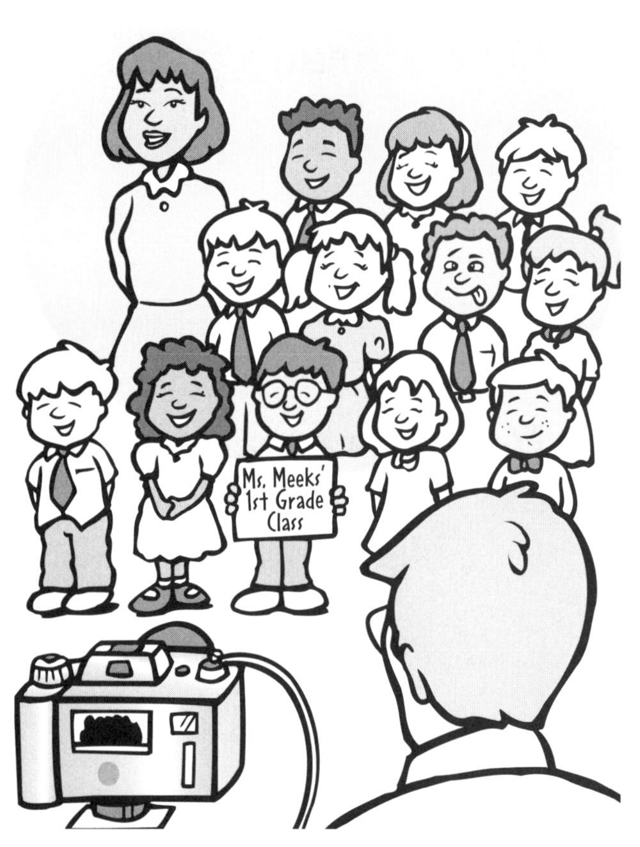

- ***Who*** takes the school picture?
- ***What*** are the children doing?

- ***Where*** is the camera?
- ***When*** do the children say "cheese"?

- ***Why*** do the children wear nice clothes for the school picture?
- ***How*** will the teacher feel when she sees the picture?

Cut on dotted line

Cut on dotted line

School Store

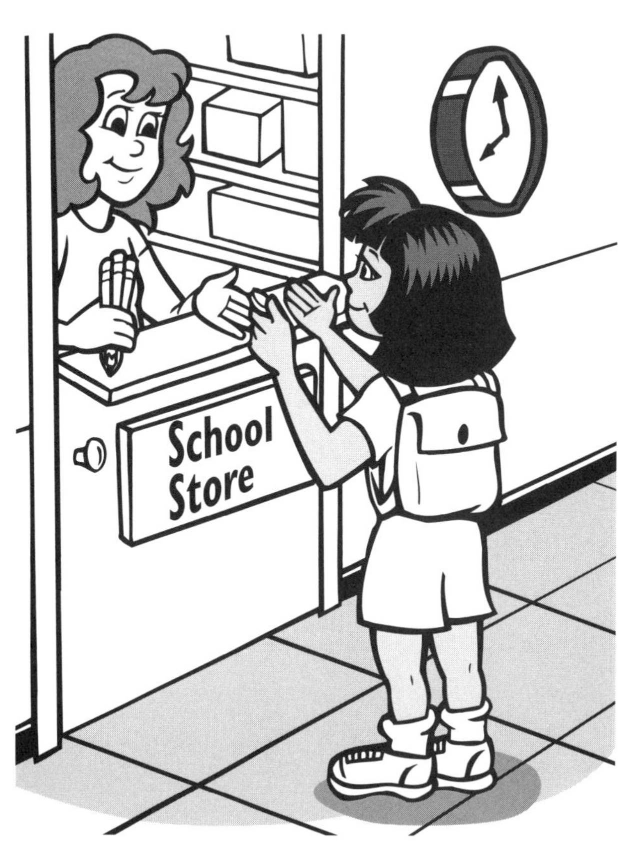

- ***Who*** is at the store?
- ***What*** is she buying?

- ***Where*** is the person selling the supplies?
- ***When*** do you buy new pencils?

- ***Why*** is the girl in a hurry?
- ***How*** do you buy something in a store?

1 2 3 4

Cut on dotted line

School

Taking a Test

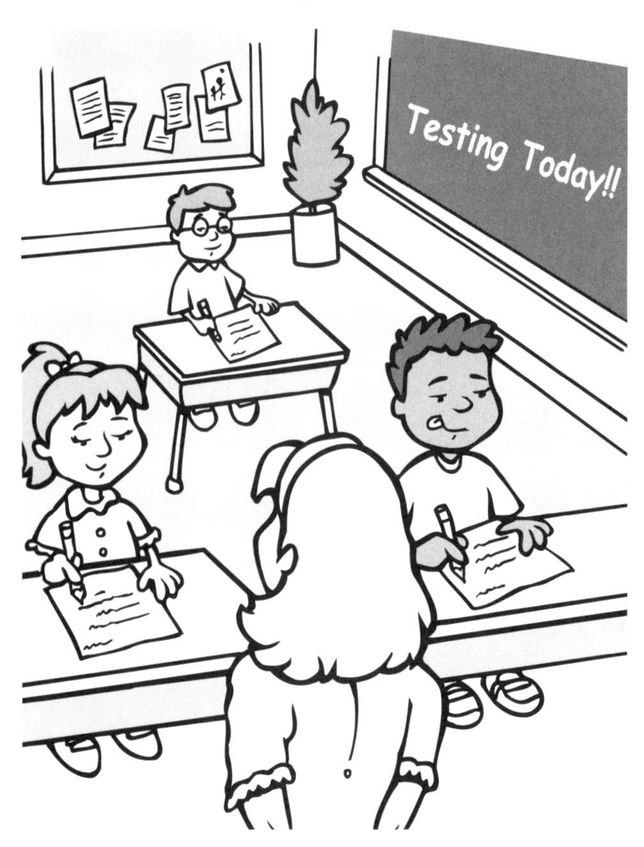

- ***Who*** is taking a test?

- ***What*** are the children using to write?

- ***Where*** are they sitting?

- ***When*** should a student study for a test?

- ***Why*** do teachers give tests?

- ***How*** do you know the children are taking a test?

Cut on dotted line

1 2
4 3

Teacher at the Chalkboard

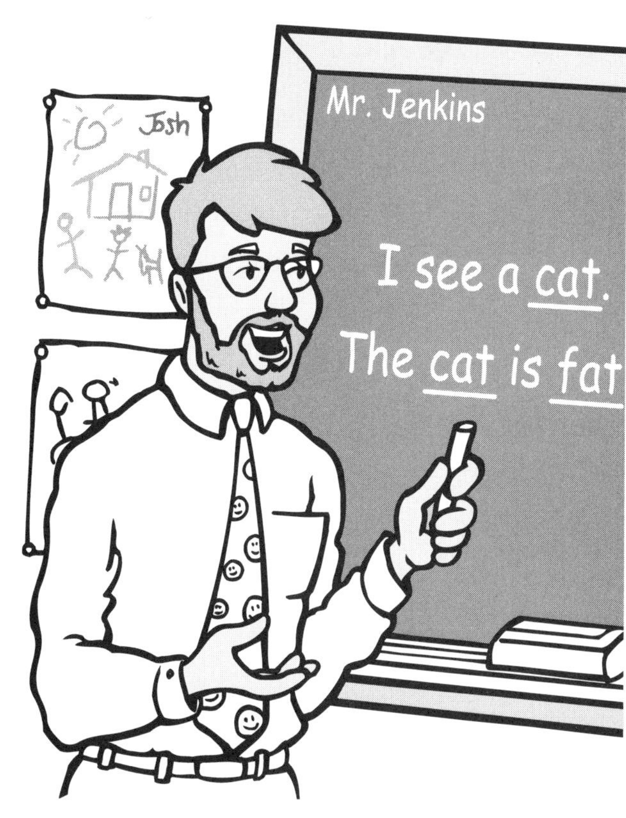
Mr. Jenkins
I see a cat.
The cat is fat
Josh

- ***Who*** is in charge of a classroom?
- ***What*** is the teacher holding?

- ***Where*** are teachers found in a school?
- ***When*** do teachers need a substitute?

- ***Why*** do teachers write on a chalkboard?
- ***How*** many different teachers have you had?

www.superduperinc.com • #BK-276

Walking to School

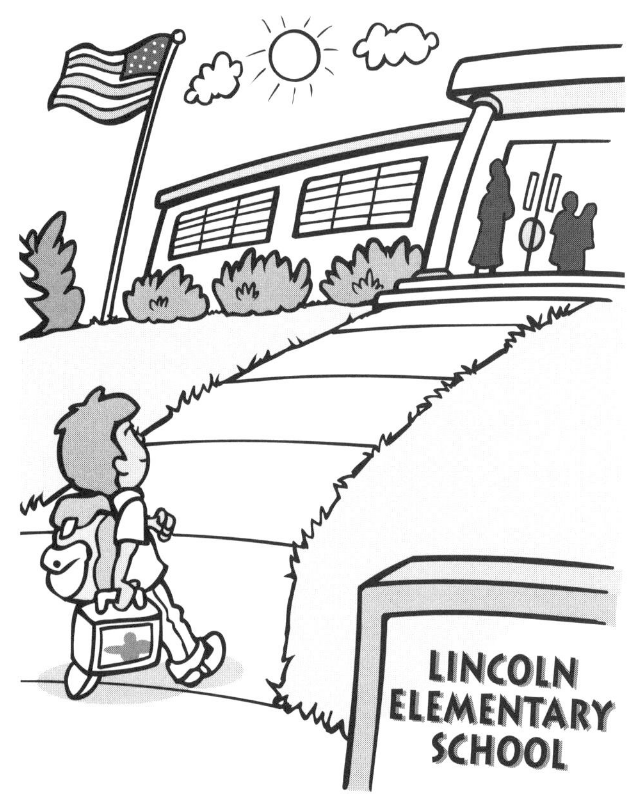

- ***Who*** goes to school?
- ***What*** do children carry to school?
- ***Where*** is the flag?
- ***When*** is there no school?
- ***Why*** is the boy wearing a backpack?
- ***How*** will the boy get home?

1 2 3 4

Cut on dotted line

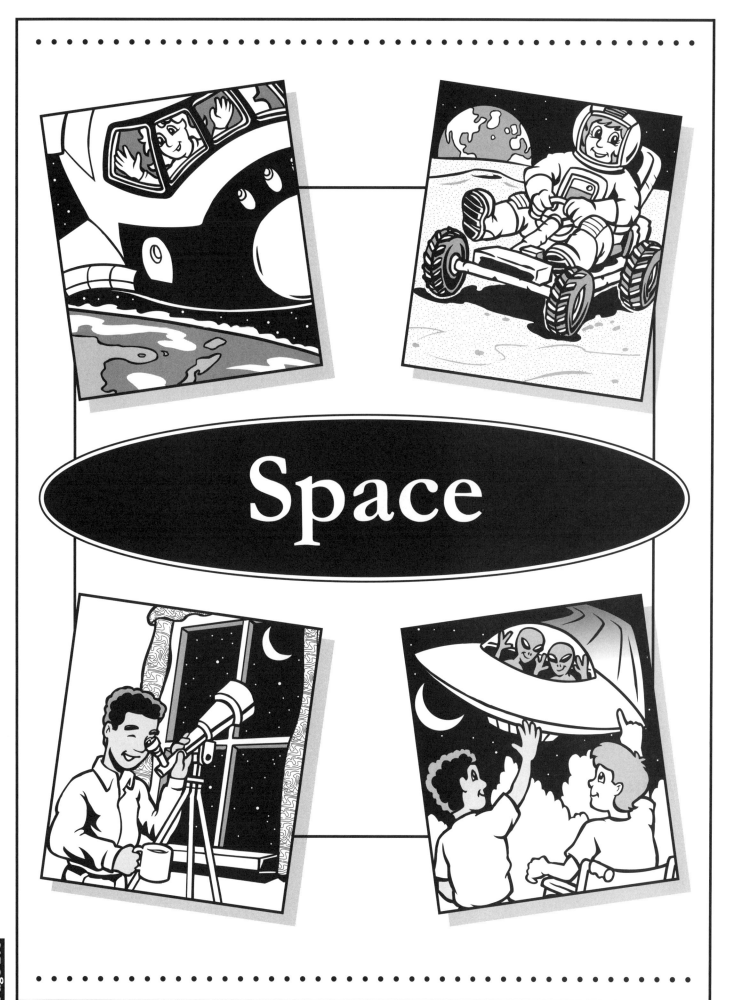
Space

Aliens Playing Cards

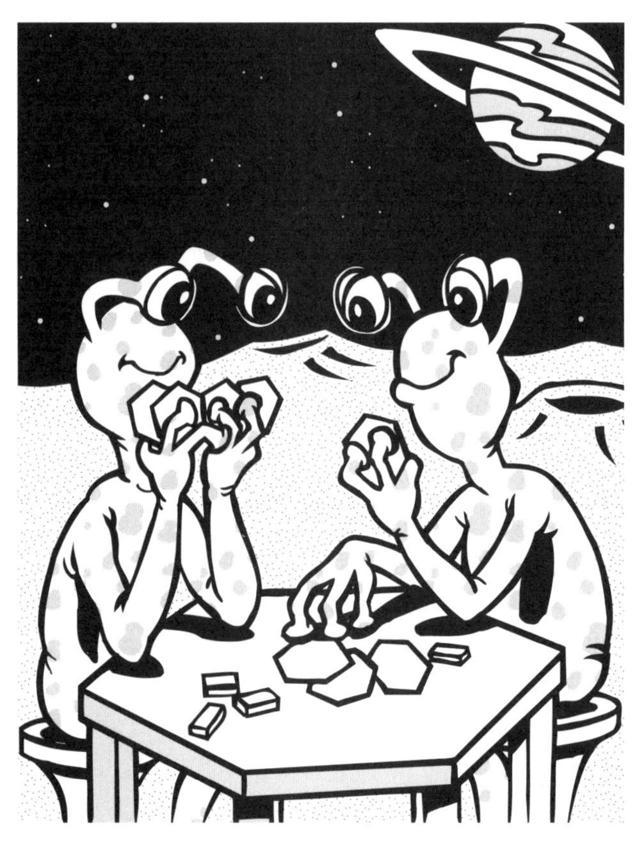

- ***Who*** is playing the game?
- ***What*** do they have in their hands?
- ***Where*** are their eyes?
- ***When*** do you get to play cards?
- ***Why*** do people and aliens like to play games?
- ***How*** do you play "Go Fish"?

Cut on dotted line

Cut on dotted line

Flying in Space

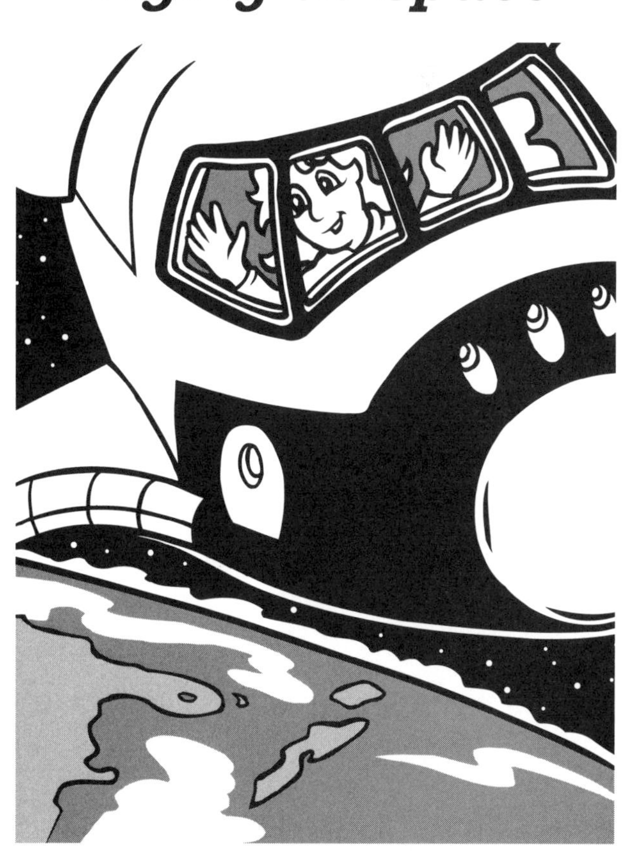

- ***Who*** is on the space shuttle?
- ***What*** is she looking at?

- ***Where*** is the Earth?
- ***When*** will she return to Earth?

1 2 3 4

- ***Why*** is she happy?
- ***How*** does the Earth look from space?

Cut on dotted line

Space

Flying Saucer

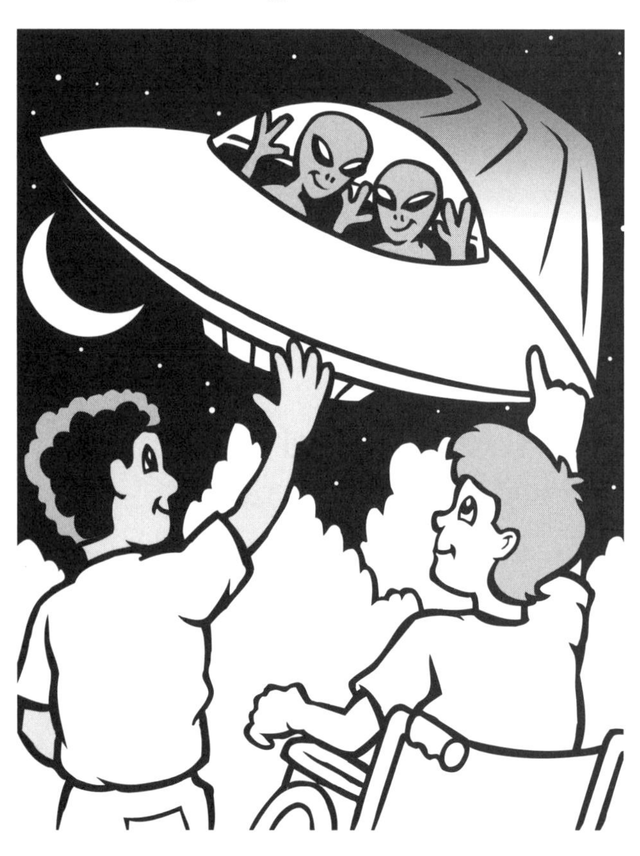

1

2

- ***Who*** sees the spaceship in the sky?
- ***What*** is the shape of the flying saucer?

3

- ***Where*** do aliens live?
- ***When*** would you see a flying saucer?

4

- ***Why*** are the boys watching the spaceship?
- ***How*** do the boys feel?

Space Shuttle

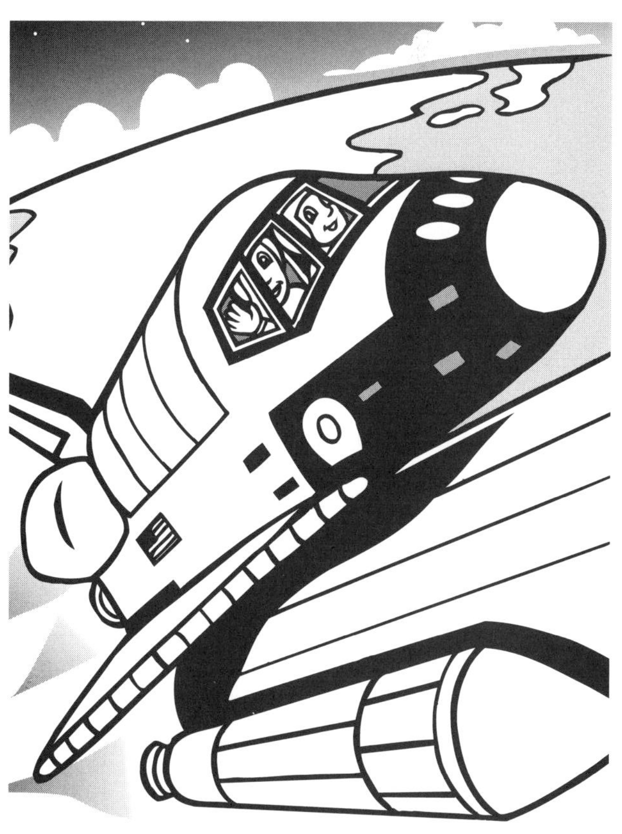

- ***Who*** flies the space shuttle?
- ***What*** is coming out of the bottom of the shuttle?
- ***Where*** are the astronauts going?
- ***When*** did they blast off?
- ***Why*** does the space shuttle have a big gas tank?
- ***How*** will the astronauts come back down to Earth?

1 2 3 4

Cut on dotted line

Cut on dotted line

1 2 3 4

Space Station

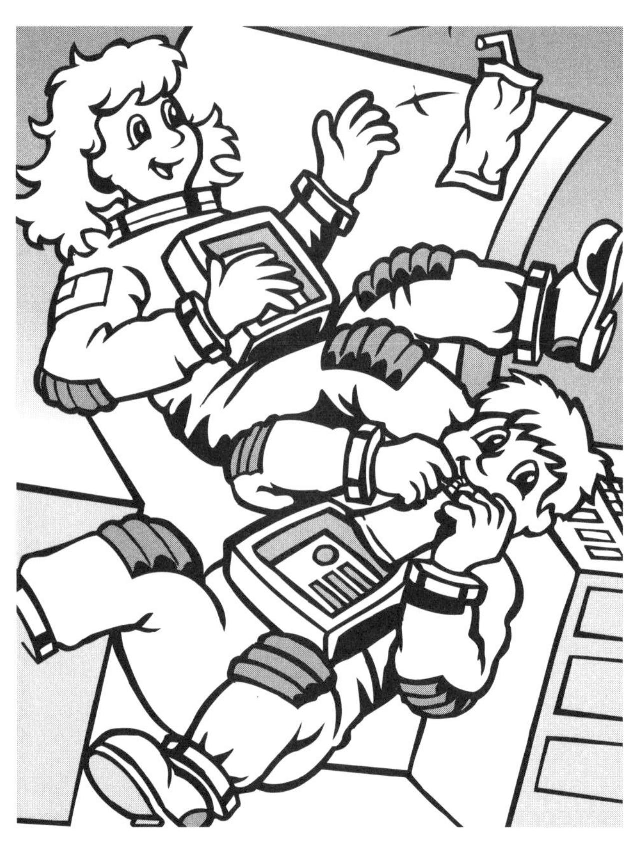

- ***Who*** is eating in space?
- ***What*** are they eating?

- ***Where*** did they get the food?
- ***When*** do you eat?

- ***Why*** is the food packet floating?
- ***How*** does this food taste?

Telescope

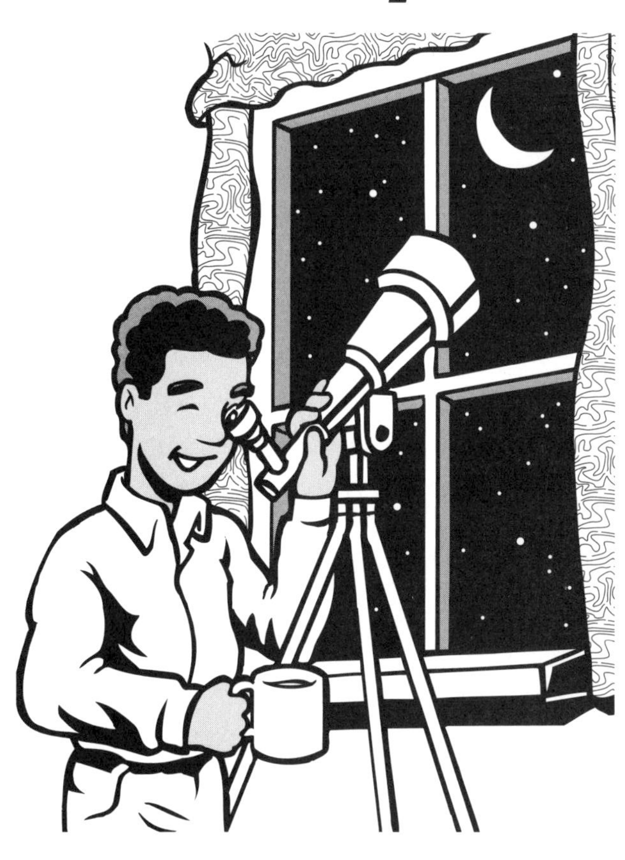

1 2 3 4

- ***Who*** is looking through the telescope?
- ***What*** does he see?

- ***Where*** is the man looking?
- ***When*** can you see the moon and stars?

- ***Why*** is the telescope so long?

- ***How*** does a person look through a telescope?

Cut on dotted line

Woman on the Moon

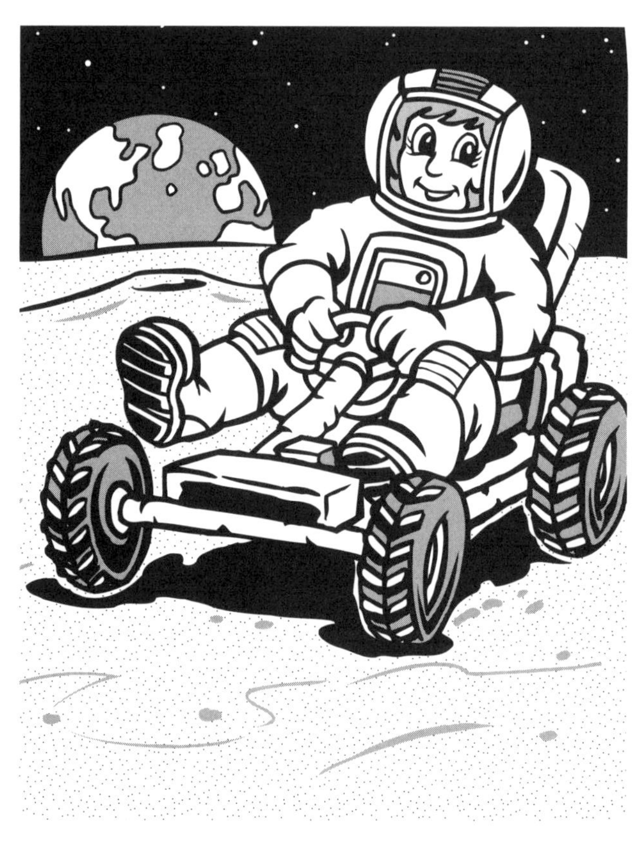

1 4
2 3

- ***Who*** is on the moon?
- ***What*** is she riding on?
- ***Where*** is she going?
- ***When*** can you see the moon from the Earth?
- ***Why*** is she wearing a space suit?
- ***How*** does a person get to the moon?

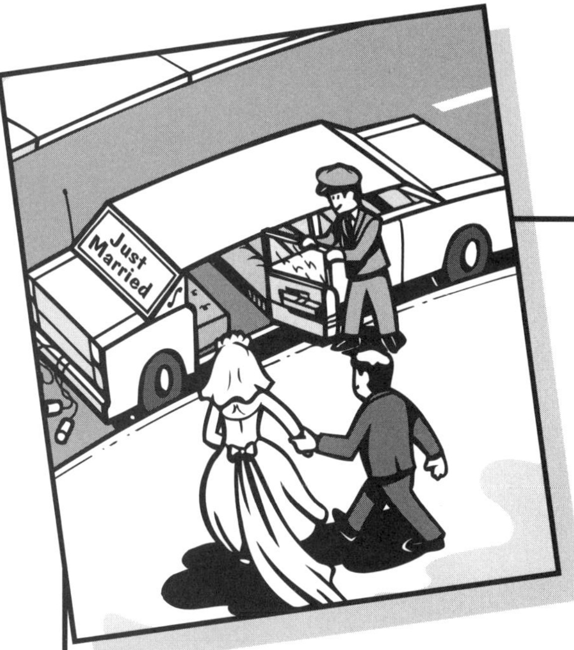

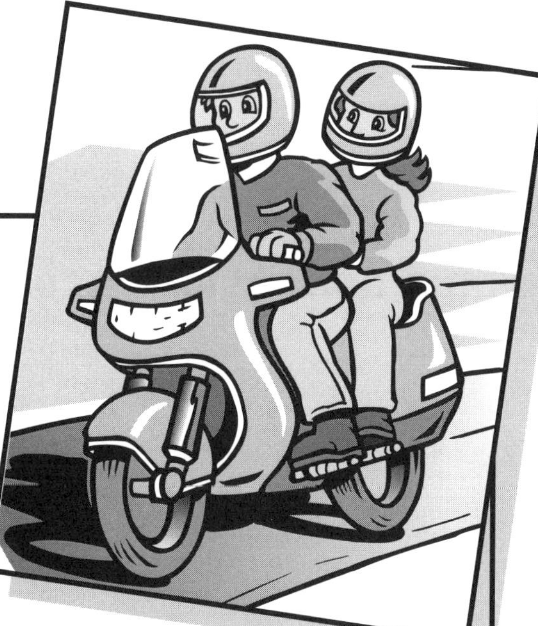

Transportation

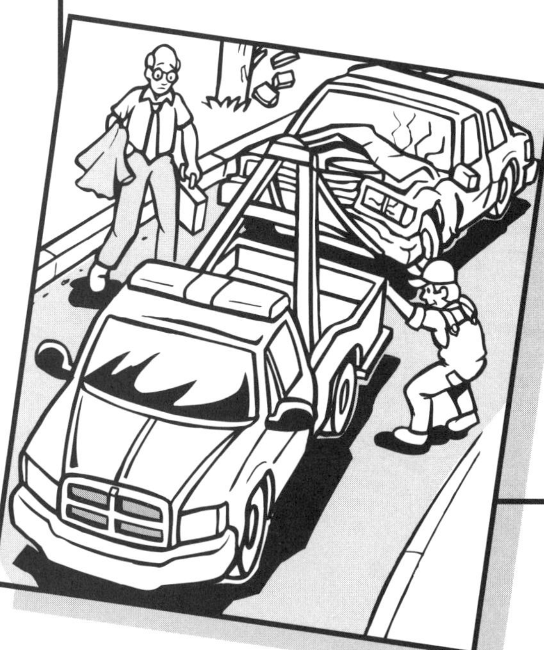

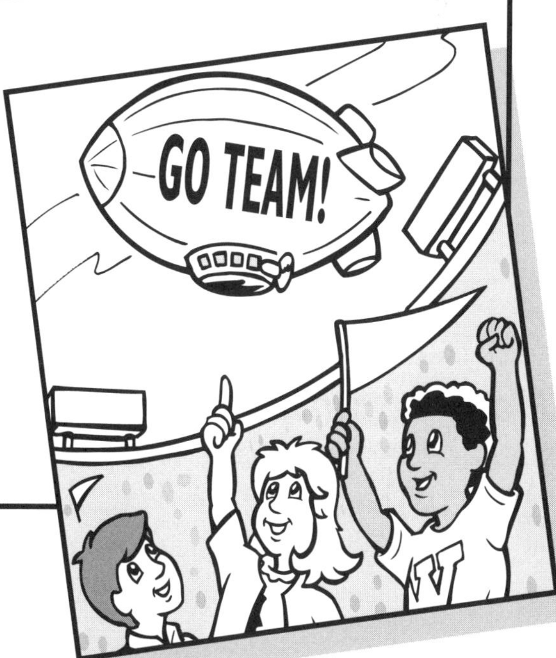

Cut on dotted line

Ambulance

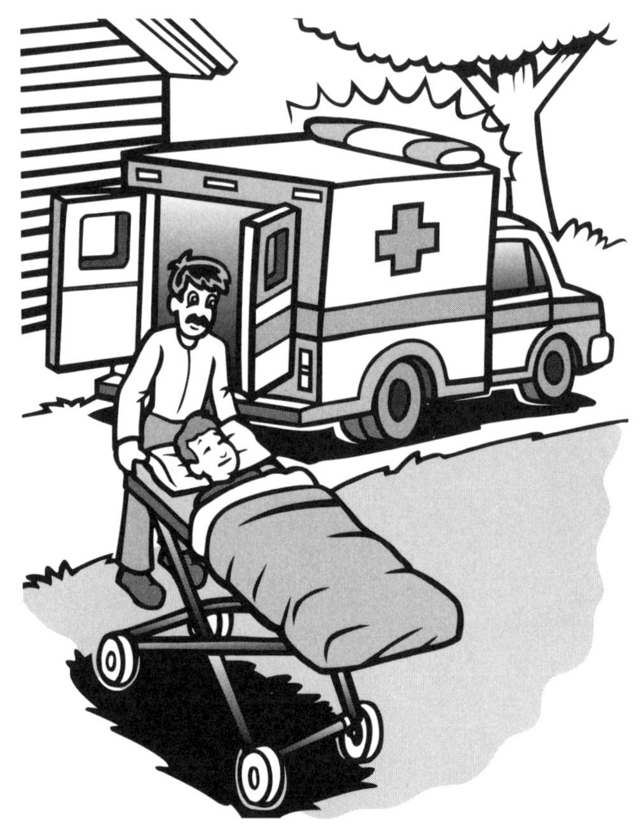

- ***Who*** is on the stretcher?

- ***What*** flashes on top of the ambulance?

- ***Where*** is the ambulance going?

- ***When*** do you call for an ambulance?

- ***Why*** do ambulances drive fast?

- ***How*** do ambulance workers put people in the ambulance?

Cut on dotted line

Blimp

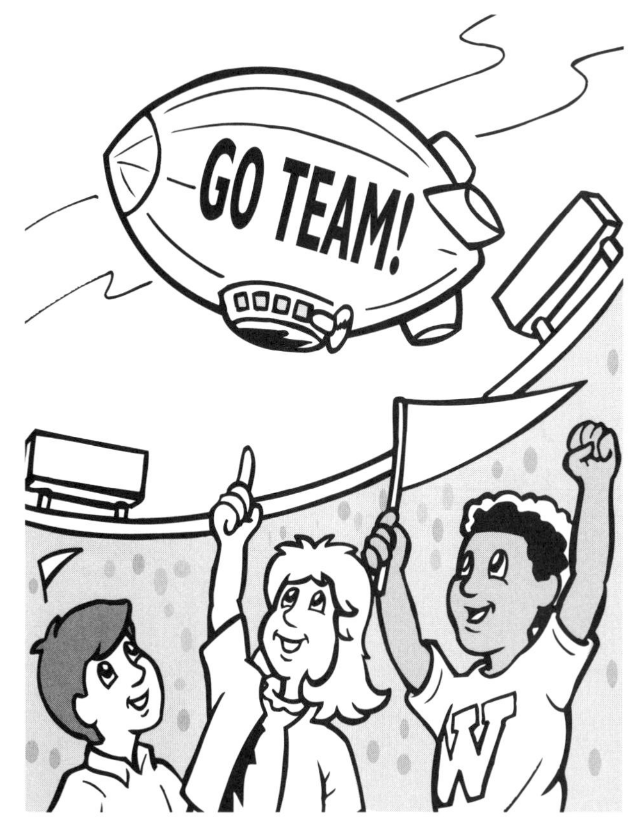

1 2 3 4

- ***Who*** is looking at the blimp?
- ***What*** shape is the blimp?

- ***Where*** else would you see a blimp?
- ***When*** will the blimp land?

- ***Why*** does the bottom have lights on it?
- ***How*** does the blimp fly?

Hot Air Balloon

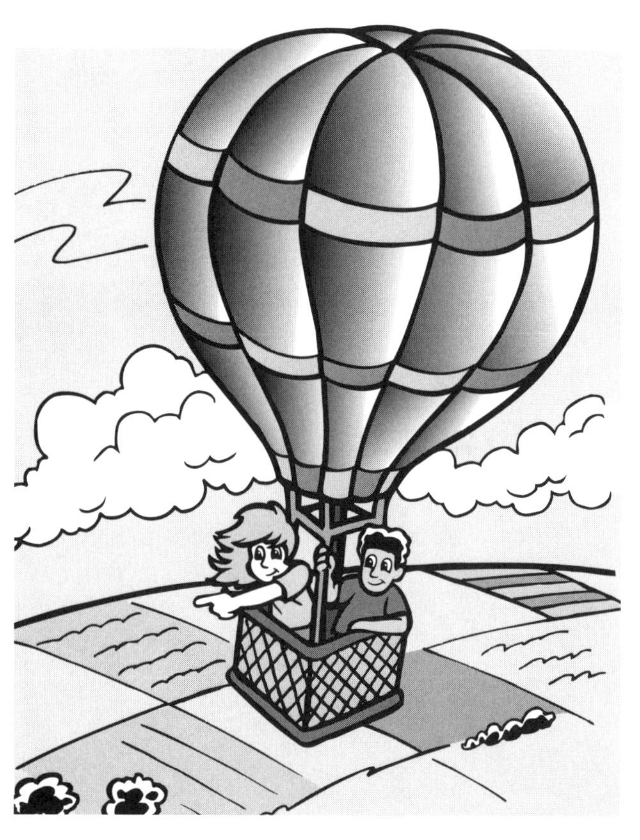

- ***Who*** is in the balloon?
- ***What*** is below the balloon?

- ***Where*** will the balloon land?
- ***When*** will the balloon need more air?

- ***Why*** do balloons have baskets underneath them?
- ***How*** does the balloon go up into the air?

Cut on dotted line

Limousine

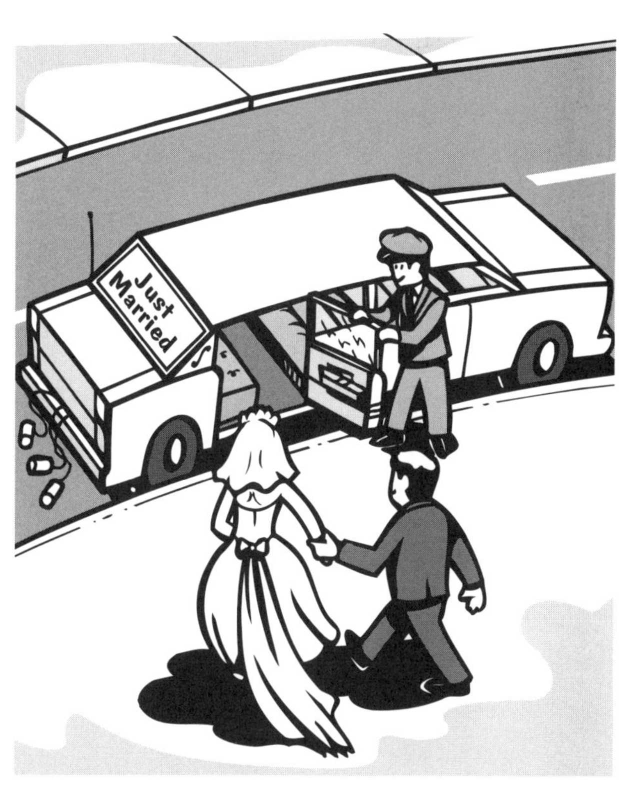

- ***Who*** drives this long car?
- ***What*** do you call this special car?

- ***Where*** will the couple ride?
- ***When*** do people ride in a limousine?

- ***Why*** do people ride in this?
- ***How*** is this vehicle different than a car?

Motorcycle

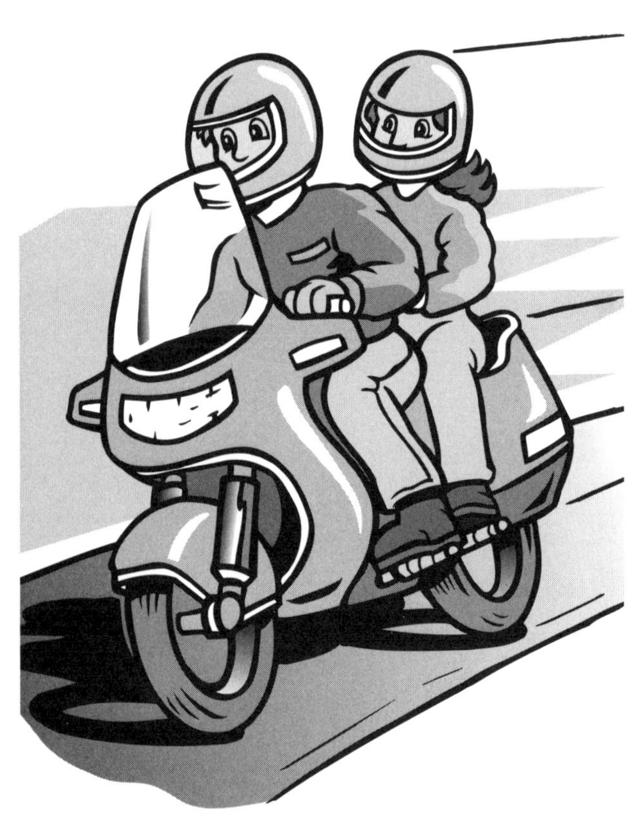

- ***Who*** is driving the motorcycle?
- ***What*** are they looking at?

- ***Where*** do people put their feet when they ride a motorcycle?
- ***When*** do people ride motorcycles?

- ***Why*** are they wearing helmets?
- ***How*** does the driver steer the motorcycle?

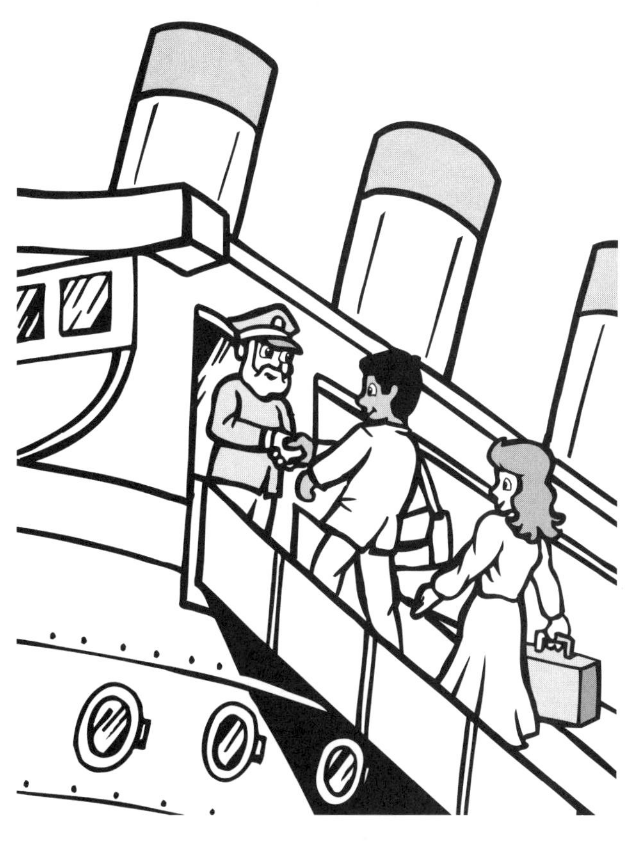

- ***Who*** is shaking hands with the passengers?
- ***What*** are these people carrying?

- ***Where*** are the people going?
- ***When*** do ships dock in a port?

- ***Why*** do people take suitcases on a trip?
- ***How*** do people get on and off the ship?

1 2 3 4

Tow Truck

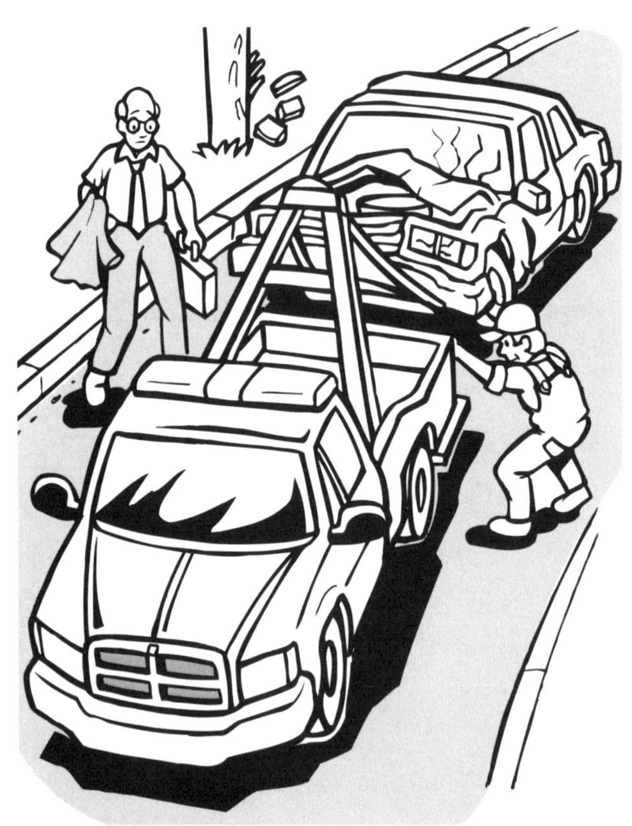

- ***Who*** drives a tow truck?
- ***What*** is the man carrying?
- ***Where*** will the tow truck take the car?
- ***When*** will the man get his car back?
- ***Why*** does the man need a tow truck?
- ***How*** did the car get wrecked?

1 2 3 4

Cut on dotted line

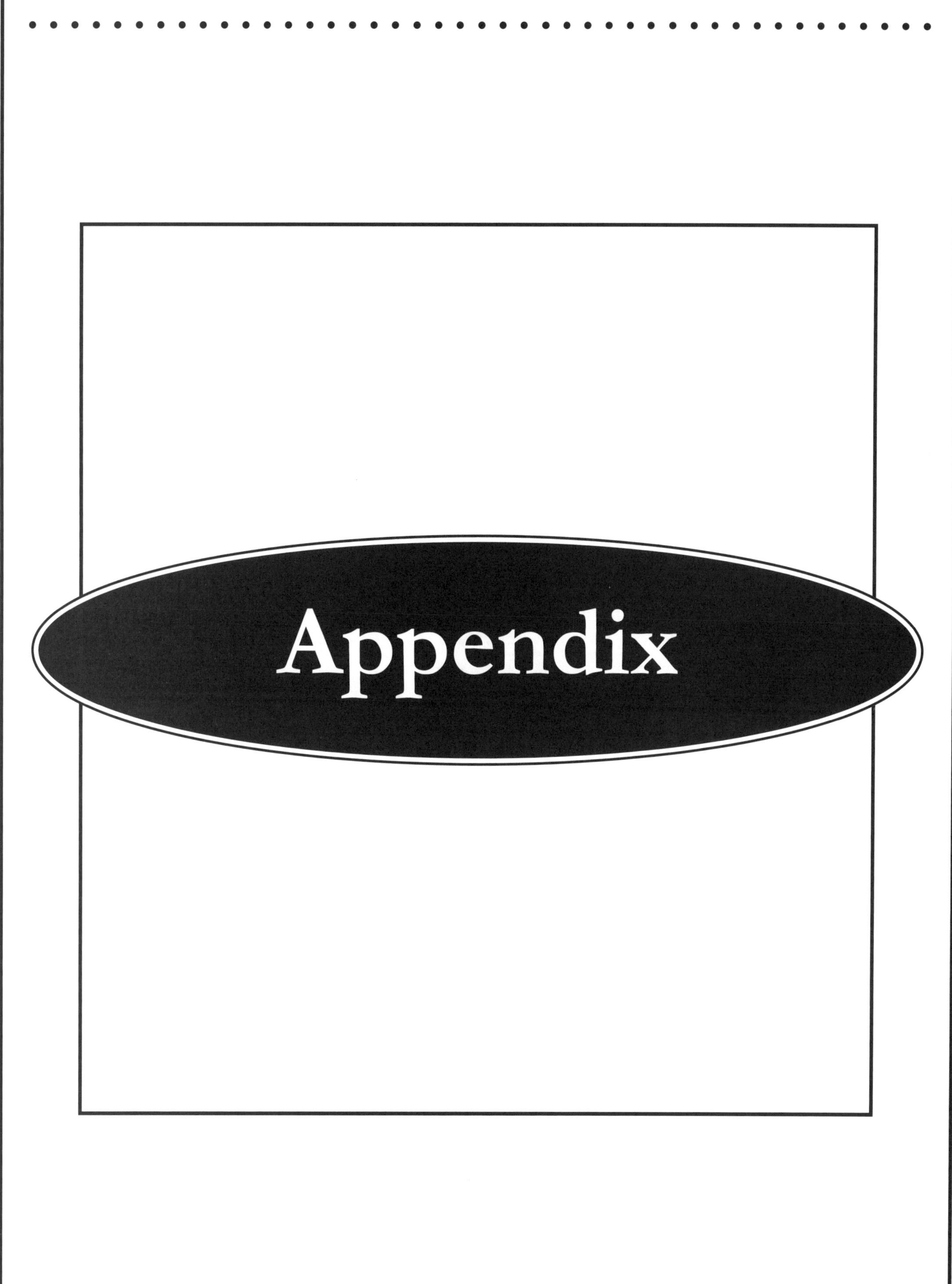
Appendix

• When

• What

• Where

• Who

3 2

4 1

• Why

• How

Cut on dotted line

Index

Notes

Notes